WHAT TO DO W.....
COLLEGE IS NOT THE BEST
TIME OF YOUR LIFE

David Leibow, M.D.

COLUMBIA UNIVERSITY PRESS   NEW YORK

COLUMBIA UNIVERSITY PRESS

Publishers Since 1893

NEW YORK   CHICHESTER, WEST SUSSEX

All patients described or referred to in this book are fictional composites
and do not correspond to any real individual.

Library of Congress Cataloging-in-Publication Data
Leibow, David.
What to do when college is not the best time of your life / David Leibow, M.D.
p.   c.m.
Includes index.
ISBN 978-0-231-15174-0 (cloth: alk. paper)—ISBN 978-0-231-15175-7 (pbk.: alk. paper)
1. College students—Mental health.   2. Counseling in higher education.   I. Title.
RC451.4.S7L45   2010
616.8900835—dc22
2009051479

Casebound editions of Columbia University Press books are printed on permanent
and durable acid-free paper.

Printed in the United States of America

c 10 9 8 7 6 5 4 3 2 1
p 10 9 8 7 6 5 4 3 2 1

For my parents, Barbara and Kevey,
my wife, Sandra,
and my daughters, Emily and Nicole.

CONTENTS

QUESTIONNAIRE:

Is What to Do When College Is Not The Best Time of Your Life *for You?*

Put a check mark beside each question you answer "yes" to. Be honest. This questionnaire isn't meant to make you feel bad about yourself. And it isn't designed to trick you into feeling negatively about college. It's designed to help you clarify whether you're having the college experience you hoped for—and that you still *could* have if you made a few changes.

GENERAL

1. Is college a disappointment? Is it less fulfilling or fun than you thought it would be?
2. Are you having more trouble fitting in or getting adjusted than you expected?
3. Do you think about transferring or dropping out?
4. Do you feel you're not ready to be in college or in *this* college?
5. Do you feel lost, confused, overwhelmed, stressed out, or sad a lot of the time?
6. Do you get anxious or depressed when you think of returning to college at the end of a vacation or visit home?
7. Does it seem as though everyone else is enjoying college more and adjusting to it better than you are?

HOMESICKNESS

1. Are you missing your parents, old friends, and home more than you expected?
2. Do you go home instead of staying on campus more than once or twice a term?
3. Are you picking fights with your parents over minor issues?
4. Do you always feel depressed or irritated after phone calls home?
5. Do you revert to childish behaviors when you're at home?
6. Are you using romantic relationships or sex to deal with loneliness?

ACADEMIC PROBLEMS

1. Is the academic work harder or more time-consuming than you expected?
2. Do you feel anxious or unbearably restless before getting down to work?
3. Does it take forever to start or complete papers?
4. Do you surf the net, watch TV, smoke pot, or just daydream to avoid doing schoolwork?
5. Do you fall asleep when you try to study or read?
6. Have you decided to make academics a lower priority than socializing?
7. Are you more than two weeks behind in your work?
8. Do you begin most assignments just before they're due?
9. Do you skip classes more than once a week?
10. Have you had incompletes at the end of the term?
11. Have you had to drop a class because you fell too far behind in the work?
12. Have you exaggerated an illness or emotional problem to get an extension?

13. Do you conceal your grades from your parents?
14. Have you changed your educational or career goals because of poor grades?
15. Are you starting to hate college because of the academic pressure?

FRIENDSHIP

1. Do you feel lonely most of the time?
2. Have you been unable to make one or two friends at college?
3. Do you feel you're a better friend to other people than they are to you?
4. Do you do favors all the time for people in order to get them to like you?
5. Do you have to drink or use drugs in order to feel comfortable socially?
6. Do you act aloof or have a chip on your shoulder to avoid rejection?
7. Do you constantly find fault with your friends or feel disappointed by them?
8. Is it hard to "be yourself" when you're with friends?

LOVE AND SEX

1. Do you think that most college students are more sexually experienced than you?
2. Do you feel uncomfortable with your sexual preference or your sexual desires?
3. Do you worry about your sexual performance or the way you look naked?
4. Are you unable to enjoy sex a lot of the time?
5. Are you attracted to partners who are rejecting or inconsiderate?

6. Do you often settle for being the confidante rather than the romantic partner of someone you like?
7. Do you avoid breaking up when you know you should?
8. Do you feel worse about yourself after spending time with your girlfriend or boyfriend?

Depression

1. Have your grades gone down because of depression or have you become depressed because you're floundering academically?
2. Do you feel depressed, sad, or blue more than once in awhile?
3. Have you become generally more pessimistic, negative, or hopeless?
4. Are you having more trouble than usual concentrating or remembering things?
5. Is it hard for you to fall asleep or stay asleep most nights?
6. Do you feel like staying in bed even after a night's sleep?
7. Have you lost your appetite or, conversely, do you compulsively overeat?
8. Is your energy abnormally low or are you worn out too easily?
9. Are you more irritable, impatient, or unsociable than usual?
10. Do you use alcohol or drugs to improve your mood?
11. Are you tormented by self-doubt, guilt, regret, or shame?
12. Do you obsess about things you should or should not have done or said?
13. Are your thoughts racing or are you too hyper to fall asleep?
14. Do you feel like life isn't worth living like this?
15. Do you have thoughts about killing yourself or wish you could die in an accident or from an illness.
16. Have you thought of ways to kill yourself or made plans to do so? IF **YES**, STOP THIS QUESTIONNAIRE AND GO TO THE STUDENT HEALTH SERVICE OR EMERGENCY ROOM—NOW!

Anxiety and Insomnia

1. Are you worried, stressed out, or anxious almost all the time?
2. Do your anxiety symptoms make you worry that something is wrong with you?
3. Do you avoid crowds or enclosed places because you're afraid of being trapped?
4. Do you get palpitations, chest pain, or tightness when you're feeling stressed?
5. Do you avoid parties or other gatherings because you feel too self-conscious?
6. Are you paralyzed by the idea of giving a presentation or talk in class?
7. Do you have trouble getting thoughts, words, or bits of music out of your head?
8. Do you have trouble sleeping most nights?

Drugs and Alcohol

1. Do you drink or smoke pot more than a couple of times a week?
2. Do you almost always drink to get drunk?
3. Do you need to get intoxicated in order to socialize?
4. Have you tried to avoid alcohol or drugs to prove you don't have a problem?
5. Do you worry that your alcohol or drug use might have gotten out of hand?
6. Have you missed classes, injured yourself, gotten into fights, blacked out, engaged in reckless sex, or driven a car after drinking?
7. Do you use cocaine or hallucinogens regularly?
8. Have you ever used methamphetamine, opiates, ecstasy, or other "hard" drugs?

9. Do you use medical or psychiatric drugs to get high?
10. Do you routinely use other students' stimulants to study or cram for exams?

Body Image, Eating Disorders, and Self-harm

1. Do you often obsess about your weight or avoid socializing because you feel fat?
2. Do you look in the mirror, pinch your stomach or thighs, and feel disgusted?
3. Do you hate the way you look?
4. Do you skip meals, cut out foods, or diet obsessively to lose weight?
5. Do you vomit or use laxatives if you feel you've eaten too much?
6. Do you use stimulants or abuse ADD medication to control your appetite?
7. Do you cut or burn yourself?
8. Do you feel more emotionally alive when you inflict pain or injury on yourself?

After you've finished the questionnaire, add up the check marks, and write down your total score and your score for each section.

If your total score is at least 10 or your score in any section is at least 3—welcome to *What to Do When College Is Not the Best Time of Your Life!* You're one of the many students for whom college sometimes (or frequently) sucks. Don't be embarrassed: you're in good company. And don't give up. *What to Do When College Is Not the Best Time of Your Life* can help you turn things around. It will help you clarify why you're getting less out of college than you hoped for. It will give you suggestions on how to make things better. And it will let you know when to get expert help.

So read on. (It would be nice, of course, if you'd buy the book.)

WHAT TO DO WHEN COLLEGE IS NOT
THE BEST TIME OF YOUR LIFE

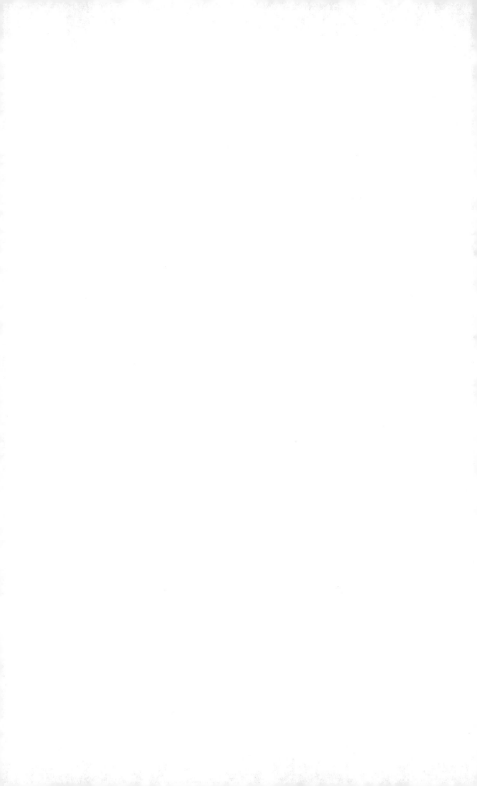

College

"The Best Time of Your Life?"

Why am I sitting motionless in front of my laptop, unable to find an opening sentence for a paper that was due yesterday, while my roommate is hitting the "send" button on a paper that's not even due until tomorrow? Why am I holed up in my tiny room on a Saturday night—eating air-popped popcorn and watching bad movies—while most of the kids on my floor are out at frat parties having fun? Why are my friends able to sing in a capella groups, write for the student newspaper, tutor local school kids, or do research, while I can barely get myself out of bed before noon? Why is everyone else slim, stylish, and dating a theater major while I'm suffering a flair-up of acne, sneak-eating junk food and playing alternate reality games on line? Why are *they* sailing happily through college while *I'm* bailing furiously just to keep from sinking?

It wasn't supposed to be this way. College was supposed to be fun. I knew it would take time to get adjusted. I knew I'd have my ups and downs. But this is way harder than I thought it would be. Everyone told me "college is the best time of your life." Either they were lying or I'm a loser!

OK, maybe I exaggerate. It's not totally terrible. I've made a few friends. A couple of my classes seem pretty interesting. The cafeteria has unlimited frozen yogurt—which is good as long as I don't gain fifteen pounds. I'm nailing Guitar Hero. And my bed *is* extralong.

It's just that everyone else seems to be living the dream. College really *does* seem to be the best time of their lives.

Meantime, I'm kind of struggling. Not that anyone can tell. I'm always cheerful and friendly. I try to sound upbeat when I talk to my parents—I don't want them to worry. But I'm not myself. I'm having trouble keeping up with my work. I procrastinate like crazy. I don't feel really close to anyone. I can't fall asleep; then I can't get up. (I've missed my 8:00 A.M. class for three weeks running.) I haven't done laundry in over a month . . .

To put it succinctly: if *this* is supposed to be The Best Time of Your Life—I don't even want to know what adulthood will be like.

In truth, the best time of your life ought to be the moment you're living in *right now*. The present, after all, is the only time you're guaranteed to have and the only time over which you have any real control. So college is not a privileged time, free of all struggle and unhappiness. It is a time like any other time—a mixture of good and bad.

Still, college is widely regarded as *among* the best times of your life. And it's understandable why this should be so: during the college years you're young and generally healthy, you're free of the direct supervision of your parents and teachers, and you have many of the freedoms of adulthood with few of the responsibilities.

Which makes it all the more shocking when college turns out to be lonely, stressful, and confusing. You were expecting cheerful, pleasant days, full of blue skies and warm sunshine. Instead you're getting too many cold, dreary days, full of fog and sleet.

One reason college enjoys the reputation for being the best time of your life is that adults tend to look back on their own college experience through a golden haze of nostalgia. They forget all the struggles and disappointments and remember only the fellowship and fun. The other reason college is viewed as exceptional is that, like you, your fellow students tend to keep their unhappiness to themselves. They put on a happy face and go about their business without revealing how they're feeling inside.

Many of your fellow students go to the student counseling service or to private psychiatrists; they just don't tell you about it. Which is a shame. Because it's hard not to feel abnormal when you don't know what normal is. Of course, it would be helpful if people were more open about what they really felt and thought. But, since no one wants to appear weak or inadequate, it's unlikely that a wave of honesty will sweep your campus anytime soon.

What to Do When College Is Not the Best Time of Your Life is designed to fill in the blanks. It describes what college students *actually* experience, the problems they commonly have, and how best to deal with those problems. In addition to standard psychiatric issues, such as insomnia, depression, and the obsession with feeling fat, *What to Do When College Is Not the Best Time of Your Life* also covers academic problems, homesickness, and the challenges of friendship and love.

The purpose of *What to Do When College Is Not the Best Time of Your Life* is to help you make college—*your* here and now—"the best time of your life" (so far).

Homesickness

TWO OF THE GLORIOUS THINGS about college are 1. the opportunity to acquire life-changing knowledge from experts who've spent their careers studying their subjects and 2. the chance to move away from home and live with people your own age. Two of the biggest adjustments required by college are 1. trying to succeed academically in a rigorous environment and 2. trying to separate from your parents and high school friends and make a home for yourself at school.

In the next chapter, I will discuss how easy it is to run aground academically. In this chapter, I want to discuss how hard it can be to make a home for yourself at school.

TWO STEPS FORWARD, ONE STEP BACK

All human desire is riddled with contradiction: I want to eat two pints of cookie-dough ice cream but I want to stay slim so I look good in jeans. I want to outscore my best friend on the LSAT, but I want to be a generous person and root for her success as well. In the developmental sphere: I want to become an adult and become independent of my parents, but I want to continue to have them as a safety net and be proud of me too.

As a college-bound student, you understand that separating from your parents is necessary for becoming adult. But that doesn't mean you're totally comfortable with the reality of doing so, or that a part of you doesn't want to stay in your old familiar surroundings—sleeping in your own bed, playing with the family pet, and having your meals prepared, your laundry done, and your wellbeing monitored by your parents.

At each stage of psychological development, the urge to grow up is met with an opposing, though weaker, desire to stay a kid. And because this desire to stay a kid is the result of strong, even overwhelming, feelings—loving attachment to, and dependence on, your parents, coupled with some fear of the world and of your own ability to cope with it—these feelings are kind of embarrassing. Especially since, according to popular myth, you're supposed to be *sick* of living at home. You're supposed to *resent* your parents and yearn for freedom.

And indeed, many college students *are* thrilled to get out of their homes and away from their parents. But if you're one of the many college students who enjoys her parents and sees them as allies, leaving the cozy world of home for the clamorous world of three-person suites, cafeteria food, and anonymous lecture halls can be more than a little bit scary.

Roz was two months into her first semester of college and still feeling homesick. She missed the quiet and solitude of her room at home. She missed walking her dog, Max. She missed lying on her parents' bed with her mother, watching their favorite TV shows. She even missed her younger brother, John, who had always been a pain in the butt.

Roz was surprised she was missing home because, during her senior year of high school, she'd been looking forward to going away to college, making a whole new group of friends and having the opportunity to become her own person. And when she first got to college she'd adjusted well: she'd met a large group of women during orientation whom she liked and who seemed to like her in return; although she had nothing in common with her roommate, they'd been pleasant to each other and figured out a routine that worked for both of them; and she'd ventured outside her comfort zone to sign up for activities, like organic farming, that were entirely new to her.

Roz had never been homesick before. She had enjoyed sleep-away camp and the one-month driving trip she'd taken across country with two friends the summer before college. She was especially surprised at feeling homesick because, when her parents had helped move her into the dorm at the end of August, she had fought with her mother nonstop. (And, truthfully, she had never walked her dog Max unless forced to.)

Roz felt ambushed and embarrassed by her homesickness and did her best to fight it. She rationed phone calls to her mother, sought out friends to have meals with so she wouldn't have to sit alone in the cafeteria, rehearsed nearly every evening with her a capella group, and created dynamite costumes for theme parties at the frats.

But one evening, watching her mother's favorite TV shows on a friend's bed piled high with stuffed animals, Roz burst into tears.

"I can't believe it," she told her friend. "I miss my mother. This is really embarrassing."

Her friend put her arms around Roz and gave her a hug. "Are you kidding?" she said. "I've gone home five times already, and it's only November!"

Like Roz, most of you will be embarrassed about feeling homesick and try to conceal it. If you were to open up to your friends a little bit, however, you'd find that homesickness is pretty common. And you'd find that it waxes and wanes with circumstances—getting worse after vacations and real or perceived social rejections, getting better after a good time with friends or a great result on an essay or exam.

For obvious reasons, homesickness is most intense during the first semester of freshman year. But it doesn't always go away completely and often flares up just before the new semester. And homesickness is not limited only to college students. In my work with single adults in their twenties and thirties who live a long way from their parents, I have been struck by how much more prone to depression they are than those who have families living nearby.

You're also not immune from homesickness just because you went away to a residential high school. Most prep schools feature a lot of adult supervision and mentoring, and the absence of that kind of adult support in college can be quite disorienting.

Homesickness is increased by other causes of unhappiness at college: academic difficulties, social disappointments, medical or psychiatric problems, and especially family problems such as divorce, illness, or death. Fortunately, it's decreased by happiness with classes, friends, and extracurricular activities.

The first symptoms of homesickness actually crop up *before* college, during senior summer. After the prom and the after-party, after graduation and the associated celebrations, after you clean out your locker for the last time, hug your friends, and say good-bye for the summer, it hits you: in three months your childhood life will be over. You'll be leaving behind the familiar routine of home and family, lifelong friends, thirteen or more years of school, old girlfriends and boyfriends, coaches and teachers, religious instruction, music lessons, your room, your bed, your pet, your parents—everything you've ever known and loved—forever. (Or so you believe.) Just thinking about it is scary.

It isn't really true, of course. You *won't* be leaving all those things behind. You won't *really* be an adult. You *will* continue to have lots of support and love. And college will probably turn out to be less daunting and more fun than you fear. Nevertheless, a certain anticipatory homesickness begins to creep in during the summer after the senior year of high school—that wonderful hiatus separating your old life from your new.

Antagonism at Home

One symptom of dawning separation anxiety is increased antagonism between you and your parents. That's part of the reason Roz and her mother fought when Roz was moving into the dorm. As if to say, *I'm not upset about your/my leaving for college, I'm actually happy about it,* hostility works both to create distance between you and your parents and deny there's any sadness connected with your leaving. It might surprise you to learn that separation anxiety affects your parents too (especially when they've already given your room to your younger brother!). But such is the case. Remember, they are "losing" their child (you) to the wider world, possibly forever.

Knowing that the antagonism between you and your parents is being caused by separation anxiety won't necessarily make it evaporate. There are two reasons for this. First, conflicts between you and your parents—especially those that arise on visits home or on vacations—will often center around apparently legitimate disagreements, such as when you should go to bed and wake up, what your duties around the house will be, and whether or not you should be required to let your parents know your plans. That these disagreements are "legitimate" disguises the fact that they're partly motivated by your mutual separation anxiety. Second, though we might wish it otherwise, antagonism between you and your parents *does* aid the process of separation. Increased conflict makes the prospect of your imminent departure seem less like a loss and more like a relief:

I can't wait to get out of here. You're driving me crazy!
We can't wait either. You've been a total pain in the neck!

The good news is: 1. You and your parents will probably declare a truce (without *actually* declaring it) a week or two before it's time for you to leave for college—although, as we've seen with Roz, tempers do tend to flare up again during move-in. 2. All hostilities will be dropped the minute you kiss your parents good-bye and drive away. 3. When you return home for a visit, you and your parents will be on your best behaviors—at least for an hour.

Regression

Another disconcerting manifestation of the evolving parent-child relationship is regression: when you're with your friends and professors you act like a grown-up; when you're with your parents you act like a kid. Regression is like reverse metamorphosis: you transform from a butterfly back into a pupa (in other words, not quite all the way back to being a caterpillar). All it takes is the sound of your mother's voice for you to crawl back into the cocoon. You go from being cheerful and confident to sullen and insecure, from self-reliant and focused to needy and disorganized. You misplace your medicine and your day-timer, drop your computer from the top bunk, forget to do your laundry until you run out of underwear, and watch TV like it was just invented. Girls call up their mothers at 3:00 A.M. crying inconsolably; boys play video games all night and sleep through their classes.

Because it seems like a step in the wrong direction, regression is embarrassing. Aren't you supposed to become *more* competent, not less, as you get older? Isn't maturation, like time itself, supposed to flow only in *one* direction—forward? Well, yes and no. The direction of maturation is not straight onward and upward; it's up and down and two steps forward, one step back.

And in this halting voyage from adolescence to adulthood, regression is a way of regrouping and renewing your resources for the next step forward. Sometimes it's nice to give yourself a little vacation from being brave and self-reliant. And sometimes—like when you're feeling utterly defeated and overwhelmed—it can't be helped. You just have to have a meltdown! (If you're a little bit considerate of your parents' feelings when you *have* your meltdown, however, you'll make it easier for them to respond appropriately.)

Falling in Love

Another traditional, and generally adaptive, way of dealing with homesickness is by falling in love. I say *generally* adaptive because, while falling in love is wonderful, the too-desperate search for a boyfriend or girlfriend can lead to bad choices. Using *romantic* love as a substitute for *parental* love is chancy. You could be lucky and find a stable and nurturing partner. But you could also be unlucky and end up in an intense and stormy relationship that is not only damaging in itself, but interferes with schoolwork and your other friendships.

Falling in love, as opposed to merely hooking up, is great. It's the all-purpose remedy for unhappiness. It makes everybody happy (until it blows up, of course). And since being "in love" is so all-consuming and confers so much cachet, it can be used to justify virtually any behavior, good or bad.

Every other responsibility or duty pales in comparison to the obligations of love. It is everyone's number one priority: *Who cares about something trivial like neuroscience? I'm in love!* And love has its own topsy-turvy logic: *How can you expect me to study Freud when my boyfriend is angry at his father and needs my understanding?*

Being part of a couple also implies maturity. Having a boyfriend or girlfriend places you on an equal footing, so to speak, with other adult couples, including your parents. You've solved the problem of homesickness by becoming an instant adult and creating your own home.

Joan was a junior at a small college in rural New England when she met Bill, a local veterinarian, at a bar in town. Bill was thirty-two years old, divorced, with a ten-year-old son who lived with Bill's ex-girlfriend, the boy's mother.

Both Joan and Bill were a little tipsy when they met, but there was an immediate attraction and, at the end of the evening, Joan agreed to give Bill her number. Bill called the next day—a behavior that was unheard of among the boys Joan knew at college—and they arranged their first date for the following Saturday night.

Joan was both excited and apprehensive about her upcoming date with Bill. On one hand, she was lonely and Bill had a protective manliness that was very comforting. On the other hand, he was much older, at a different stage of life, had a lot of baggage, and, despite being a vet, had been raised in an entirely different socioeconomic background.

On their first date, Joan decided to sleep with Bill. The sex was amazing: he was a confident and considerate lover and a perfect gentleman. But the next day she decided not to see him again. She wasn't sure why. There was just something "off" about him. He drank too much, lacked sophistication, and his charm felt manipulative.

Bill called again the day after the date. They had a pleasant conversation, but, when he asked Joan out, she made an excuse about exams and papers and said she couldn't go.

Bill called again the next day and the day after and the day after that—until Joan finally agreed to a second date. Why? Because she was lonely and he was cute and because—unlike the college boys who played games and never showed sustained interest in her—Bill really, really seemed to like her.

The second date was followed by a third and a fourth. Within a month, Joan had talked herself out of her reservations about Bill, and they were boyfriend and girlfriend. "He adored me," she explained.

Joan spent her last two years of college almost exclusively with Bill. She moved in with him off campus and, as a result, became increasing less involved with her friends, her academic work, and the college experience in general.

In an irony that would only become apparent to Joan much later, her relationship with her parents was strained as well. She knew they were worried about her choice of boyfriend, her slipping grades, and her increasing isolation from her friends, but she wouldn't allow them to discuss their worries with her. "You're just making me angry," she told them.

When I met with Joan after graduation she described her last two years of college as a dark time.

"I realize now that I was depressed," she told me. "I knew my parents and my friends were right about my relationship with Bill, but I kept telling myself I was in love and that love demanded sacrifice. Bill was supportive of me in a way my parents couldn't be, considering their disapproval of my choices; and he was critical of my friends for being unsupportive. He acted like he was my only supporter, which, in retrospect, drove a further wedge between me and my parents and friends.

"Bill constantly flattered me, which I felt I needed," she explained. "At the same time, he drank too much, he had a wicked temper, and I could see from the way he and his ex-girlfriend were raising their son that we had very different ideas about child rearing.

We had very different upbringings too: He was alienated from his parents, who were disgustingly stingy and mean, whereas I was—or used to be—close to my parents, who were unbelievably generous and loving."

With tears in her eyes, Joan explained that she had tried to break up with Bill on many occasions but had been unable to do so. "I looked for excuses—like when he drank too much or was nasty to me—but he kept talking me into staying. He'd cry and plead and tell me I was the only thing good in his life. I didn't know how to get out of it without hurting him or making him scary-angry. I was a little afraid that, if I left him, he'd hurt himself or me. The worst part was I was too ashamed to tell my parents that I felt trapped."

Feeling unable to get help from her parents, Joan wisely decided to see a therapist in the town where she was attending college. (She was too embarrassed to go the college counseling service—a mistake—but that's another matter.) The advice the therapist gave her, however, was less than helpful. Instead of respecting Joan's appropriate doubts about the relationship and helping her gain the courage to end it, the therapist told Joan that her real problem was her inability to stand up to her parents. "She said my parents had undermined my independence by being unsupportive of my decision to live with Bill. When I told the therapist I understood why my parents felt the way they did about the relationship, and that I knew they were expressing their opinion out of love and concern, she took that as proof that I was still too influenced by them."

Joan concluded her account by telling me how she was finally able to extricate herself from the relationship. "Bill wanted me to stay and work in town after graduation. Luckily, I had the excuse that I was an art history major and had to get a job at a museum or gallery in the city. He offered to move here with me but, because he specializes in large animals, he couldn't find a position."

Half a year later, Bill was still calling and texting Joan, sending her e-mails and leaving messages on Facebook (because she was afraid to unfriend him). And, even though she was reconnecting with old friends, enjoying her work at a gallery, and happy to be on good terms with her parents, Joan was still feeling guilty and sad about having hurt him.

There is nothing wrong, of course, with having a boyfriend or girlfriend in college. And there's probably not much wrong with using that relationship as a way of coping with loneliness and homesickness. Millions of people become couples for just that reason. What you don't want to do is use the relationship to escape from the necessary process of becoming independent and self-reliant. And you don't want to shirk your duty to yourself to have the total college experience—to make new friends, participate in campus life, and successfully complete your academic work.

In fact, the *best* way to cope with homesickness is just that—to have the total college experience: to make new friends, participate in campus life, and successfully complete your academic work.

Another way to help cope with homesickness is to spend some time with adults. Every college catalog will tell you to contact your professors to discuss academic questions and make the learning process more personal. This is excellent advice—but for more than academic reasons. True grown-ups are as rare on college campuses (especially nonurban campuses) as young people are in nursing homes. Forming a relationship with a friendly professor, dean, adviser, or coach can help correct the maturity deficit and make you feel more at home.

Making a visit home is a complicated business. Looking forward to it, making the outgoing trip, and spending the first day with your parents are usually pretty enjoyable. Preparing to go back to school, making the return voyage, and saying good-bye—not so enjoyable. It gets better once you're back at school for a few hours, but it's always an adjustment.

Sometimes the morale boost of going home is erased by the angst of coming back. This is definitely the case if going home causes you to fall behind in your schoolwork. (Mind you, is there anyone who hasn't lugged twenty pounds of books home, full of good intentions, only to lug them back unopened? I don't think so.)

Like Roz's roommate, who went home five times in the first two months of college, you should use your own judgment about when to go home. Going home too often may prolong the adjustment to college, but not going home enough will make it unnecessarily harsh. If you're uncertain about how much to go home, it's probably better to err on the side of too much rather than too little. Having control over when you go home reduces the feeling of urgency about having to do so.

Dealing With Your Parents Once You're Over the Homesickness Hump

Titrating how much you want your parents to be involved with you when you're away at college requires ongoing assessment and adjustment. Sometimes you'll want to reach out to your parents (and be hurt they haven't made more of an effort to reach out to you). Sometimes you'll want them to give you space (and be abrupt with them when they call to inquire how you're doing). It often seems as though neither they nor you can get the distance exactly right.

In most cases, your parents will take their cue from you: If you act mysterious or give vague and defensive answers to their questions about your welfare, they'll worry about you and become more intrusive; if you act friendly and upbeat, they'll assume things are OK and become more relaxed. Their faith in you and their willingness to let you make decisions on your own will increase—or ought to—as they witness the growth of your maturity and judgment over the four years of college.

Staying Close to Home

One obvious solution to the problem of homesickness is to stay close to home—to attend college in your hometown or in a nearby town. Of course, you might *have* to stay close to home out of necessity—because of financial constraints or family obligations. There's no reason you can't have a terrific college experience living at home, provided you put in the effort to make new friends and get involved in on-campus activities.

If you have the option of attending college away from home but are worried you might be too homesick to enjoy it, you have an important decision to make. And there's no one answer that's right for everyone. It's true that living in a dorm (which you can do even in your own hometown) without the comforts of home, fending for yourself without the supervision of your parents, and overcoming homesickness all foster self-reliance and autonomy. But so does spending most of the day on campus, coping with the academic challenges of college, and getting four years older.

We all develop at our own pace and we each have a different psychological makeup. Maybe you started reading at the beginning of first grade, maybe at the end. Did it really make a difference? If you honestly believe that living far from home will make your college experience miserable, don't do it. Life is long. Once you're ready, leaving home will be easy.

(And there's a good chance you're going to end up living in your parents' basement after college anyhow!)

Academic Problems

You're walking down a corridor to a classroom where you're about to take an exam. The corridor is filled with unfamiliar students waiting to be let into the exam room. They're poring over their notebooks.

You enter the exam room and take your seat. A teaching assistant hands out the tests and exam books and chalks the start and stop times on the blackboard. All around you students are furiously writing. Except for the scraping of chairs and the scratch of pens, the room is hushed.

You strain to decipher the exam, but the words remain indistinct, as if you were looking at them through the bottom of a water glass. Meanwhile, the time continues to tick away. A feeling of panic takes root in the center of your chest.

Calm down, you tell yourself. There's still plenty of time.

Now a new problem arises. The words seem like a foreign language. Nothing makes sense. What course is this anyway?

Then it hits you. This is Religion 666. You skipped all the classes. You did none of the reading.

You can feel your consciousness leave your body. You're looking at yourself from outside. You recognize yourself as that pathetic character, familiar from a million movies, who has trapped himself in a catastrophe of his own making.

Then you wake up.

The strange students, the blurry exam, the unfamiliar material—thank God, none of it was real.

Does this sound familiar? Exam dreams and their variants are as universal as dreams of losing your teeth or walking around without your pants. And they don't go away just because you're no longer in school. I know eighty year olds who have exam dreams. And when they wake up, they're still just as relieved as when they were eighteen. The difference is that for an eighty-year-old the exam dream can no longer become reality whereas for an eighteen or twenty-two year old in college the exam dream can become a reality at any moment. Indeed, if you're one of the thousands of college students who's skipping classes, surfing the net instead of studying, smoking too much pot, procrastinating about starting assignments, making up excuses to get extensions, or taking incompletes, the exam dream *is* your reality.

And it's no longer a dream; it's a nightmare.

Every student who wakes up from an exam dream (after enjoying his moment of relief) makes a pledge to turn over a new leaf and stay on top of his work. You will too. But if you've been dogging it since high school (or even since elementary school), you'll make the pledge, you'll take a break, and then you'll break the pledge.

In this chapter, I'm going to review some of the reasons for academic floundering in college and some of the things you can do to turn over a new leaf. At the end of the chapter I'm going to explain what to do when you *don't* turn over a new leaf.

REASONS FOR ACADEMIC FLOUNDERING IN COLLEGE

It's very easy to flounder academically in college. It's especially easy to flounder in your freshman year. The classes are either harder or easier than they were in the senior year of high school—if harder, they require more work to master; if easier, they're too easy to blow off. You spend fewer hours in the classroom and more in the lab than in high school, and many introductory courses are given in large impersonal lectures. You have to do most of the work on your own without supervision. There are more distractions and no adults around to give you encouragement or to tell you no.

The biggest reason that freshman year is harder, however, is that by the time you arrive in college many of you—you know who you are—are suffering from an advanced case of senioritis. You stopped working in December of your senior year of high school after submitting your college applications and now, nine months later, you're intellectually out of shape and academically rusty. It actually *hurts* to do schoolwork—which means that one hour of studying at the beginning of the term is more painful than three hours will be at the end.

The ideal remedy for freshman jitters would be to let college students decide before graduation whether or not they wanted to have their first-year grades appear on their transcripts and count toward their final GPAs. In the meantime, some colleges already make first-semester freshman classes "pass/no record" or make "pass/fail" an option.

Almost all universities have freshman seminars and beefed-up advising to ease the transition from high school to college. Still, academic work in college can be intimidating, especially since most of us put pressure on ourselves by trying to repeat past successes or vowing to make a fresh start.

Despite the challenges, most of you will find a way to succeed in college. Let me repeat this more succinctly: Most of you will succeed in college. You should feel confident that, if you've been able to get *into* college, you should be able to get *out* of it at the other end. And, as you advance through the years and can choose your courses more freely and knowledgeably, you'll likely do better and better.

But what if you *are* struggling academically? What if you *can't* find a method that works for you even after two or three years of college? What if you begin to flounder and can't seem to get back on track?

What You *Should* Do

Here are a couple of things you *should* do:

1. Don't panic. If you deal with your academic problems now instead of waiting until some vague time in the future, you should be able to reverse the downward trend. Unfortunately, this is precisely what most of you *don't* do. You bury your heads in the sand. You skip classes you don't feel prepared for. You put off, or quit, studying altogether and fail to turn in assignments on time or at all. Eventually you reach a point of no return. Then you're forced to take an incomplete, drop the course, or accept a low grade.

College is the beginning of adulthood. And dealing with problems is what adults do. You'll have problems throughout your life—everybody does. (And, by the way, they're just as likely to be self-inflicted in the future as your current academic problems are today.) Dealing with your academic problems now will advance you along the path to adulthood and make it easier for you to deal with more serious problems later on. So don't panic, but don't put off dealing with your problems—and becoming an adult.

2. Meet with your professor. Most professors will be helpful and understanding. They deal with floundering students all the time. And although they can't—and shouldn't—give you a pass (in either sense of the word) just because you meet with them, they *will* be more accommodating than if you show no respect by ignoring them and blowing off the class or the assignments.

Seems obvious, and yet most of you won't talk to your professors about your difficulties. Why? Two reasons: shame and pride (they're two sides of the same coin.) On the one hand, you feel embarrassed by your predicament (shame): you believe your professors will think less of you for admitting you have an academic problem. On the other hand, you feel smarter than the average student who has to work hard every day to succeed (pride): you like to believe you'll be able to pull a rabbit out of a hat, even if you start your assignments the night before the deadline.

What You *Actually* Do

What do you *actually* do instead of dealing with your academic slide? You rationalize. Instead of working, you expend your mental energy coming up with "explanations" about why you're not doing what you should be doing. The problem is, once the rationalizations begin, there is no end to them. You can almost taste the desperation in the pit of your stomach as you bs yourself trying to postpone the inevitable.

I'll salvage the course by acing the final exam, you tell yourself. *I'll write a paper that will blow the instructor's socks off. It's too late to do a good job now; I'll wait and turn in all the overdue assignments after the midterm break. Worst-case scenario: I'll take an incomplete and finish the final paper early next term.*

That's what you *tell* yourself. But what do you actually *do?* You take a break.

No use getting stressed out, you reason. *That'll paralyze me. Tomorrow morning I'll get up early and make a fresh start. I've always done my best work just before the deadline anyway. In the meantime—just for this afternoon—I'll relax a little. I'll go on a food run with my roommates, check whether my ex-girlfriend has taken my picture off Facebook, or play video games for a few hours. Maybe I'll just go back to my room and take a nap.*

You rationalize and you avoid. So the problem gets worse. Which leads to more desperate rationalization and more anxious avoidance.

Eventually, one of two things happens: you either get down to work or get very, very unhappy—first with yourself, then with college.

Of the two choices, I heartily recommend the former—getting down to work. Everyone knows it's far more effective and less stressful to work steadily from the very beginning of the term. Everyone knows it's best to start assignments early, make and review notes, visit the instructor during office hours, and study in a place where you won't be distracted or bored. But having treated and taught many students over the years, I know that the majority of you—even the most successful—procrastinate. Sometimes you procrastinate because you're busy doing nonacademic activities. More often, you procrastinate because you're anxious about starting.

The big difference between those who succeed and those who fail is that those who succeed *do* eventually start their work—and finish enough of it to get a decent grade.

Which gets us to the biggest reason students—and people in general—don't get their work done.

LAZINESS

Let me share an interesting observation with you: of all the college students who've been referred to me over the years because they were in danger of failing their semester, very few—in fact, almost none—have attributed their predicament to laziness. They'll admit to procrastination or being overscheduled. They'll say they've been socializing too much, watching too much TV, spending too much time on the Internet, or smoking too much pot. They'll wonder if they have ADD or depression. They'll cop to perfectionism or anxiety. They'll say they deliberately made their girlfriend or boyfriend a higher priority than their schoolwork. They'll say their classes bore them or point out that Bill Gates and Mark Zuckerberg never graduated college. But what they won't say is that they're lazy.

Why is that? Why does saying you're lazy sound worse than saying you spend too much time surfing the net or smoking pot? Why is laziness condemned as a moral failing (sloth) while procrastination is dismissed as a minor flaw (distractibility)—especially when you consider that they both produce exactly the same result—an absence of work? I think it's because we ascribe antisocial motives to lazy people and good intentions gone awry to procrastinators. According to conventional wisdom, lazy people are freeloaders who believe the world owes them a living, whereas procrastinators are flawed people who believe in hard work—they just have trouble getting down to it. Lazy people are entitled, whereas procrastinators are easily bored. (It should be said that most parents and professors aren't able to perceive the subtle distinction between procrastination and laziness. All *they* see is laziness!)

The problem is that contrasting laziness with procrastination (or surfing the Web, smoking pot, or watching too much TV) is a distinction without a difference—and not just because they both keep you from getting your work done. The reason there's no real difference is that lazy people and people who find other reasons to avoid doing work have the same underlying motivation: they find work unpleasant—*very* unpleasant. Students who procrastinate find work *so* unpleasant, in fact, that living with the anxiety of procrastination seems easier to bear than making their heads hurt by studying and writing papers.

Yes, there probably are some people who believe they shouldn't have to work—perhaps there are a few European aristocrats still around from the nineteenth century—but I've rarely encountered one. Most of the students I've met *want* to work. They just have great difficulty making themselves do it.

And not *all* work, either—just schoolwork, because laziness tends to be situation specific. The varsity volleyball player who can't turn in her economics assignments on time will kill herself for three hours every day at practice. The sleepy guy who can't get out of bed to attend his 11:00 A.M. class will be on the golf course ready to tee off at 6:30 every Saturday morning.

Fortunately, the miserable college student who barely manages to graduate often becomes an outstanding employee once he gets into the workforce. Why is that? Why is schoolwork harder to start and easier to stop than other compulsory activities (like varsity athletics) or equally demanding extracurricular activities (like writing for the college paper)? Why is it that, for many people, working ten hours in an office or store during the summer or after college is easier than working for two hours in the library during college?

Here's why:

In college, you're left to your own devices with large swaths of unscheduled time punctuated by periods of intense, round-the-clock, lonely exertion. At work, your time is structured, the effort more uniformly distributed, and you're generally part of a team.

In college, you're living in a group setting, there are myriad distractions, and your workday never ends. At work, you're living in your own home, you can more easily shut out distractions, and, once the workday ends, your time is usually your own.

In college, your major may have nothing to do with your career, your reward is fairly abstract (good grades), and your professor is often remote and indifferent to your performance. At work, your vocation is more likely an activity you enjoy and gained competence in, your rewards are concrete (promotions and raises), and your boss cares—a lot—about whether or not you're doing a good job.

Finally, the capacity for sustained work increases as you get older. You become *less* lazy as you mature. You can sit longer, focus better, defer gratification more easily, and deal with authority more comfortably. In other words, as you get older, work becomes less like work.

The Chicken or the Egg

One difficulty in trying to help students who are floundering academically is that the factors that produce or aggravate laziness—ADD, substance abuse, depression, etc.—can also be produced or aggravated *by* laziness. Sometimes you can't sort out whether the mental disorder is causing the academic problem or the academic problem is causing the mental disorder. In most cases, each is causing the other.

One early December morning, I received a phone call from the mother of a college junior requesting an urgent appointment for her twenty-one-year-old son, Jack, who was withdrawing from school for the rest of the semester and flying home at the end of the week.

"Jack seemed fine when he was home for Thanksgiving," his mother told me in an anguished voice. "But we just got a call from him, crying, telling us he wants to come home. He said he's stopped going to classes and is very, very depressed. I think he's also smoking a lot of pot."

Jack's mother gave me a little history over the phone: He was the eldest of three children, beloved by everyone, never moody, a great athlete, a star at summer camp where he worked as a sports instructor. "Jack is very bright," she assured me. "But he might be a little ADD—he always had a tendency to procrastinate doing assignments. Even so, he did well enough in high school to get into [an excellent state university]."

At the end of our conversation I told Jack's mother, "After a few visits, if Jack gives his consent, I would like you and your husband to attend one of his appointments. That will give you a chance to express your observations and concerns and make sure we're all on the same page." A family meeting also gives the parents a chance to check out whether the therapist treating their precious son or daughter is competent and sane!

The following week, Jack showed up for his first appointment ten minutes late. Was it ambivalence about coming to see me, a sign of disorganization due to ADD or depression, or was the subway delayed as he claimed? (Jack continued to be five or ten minutes late for many of his later appointments, typical of people with ADD.)

The first thing I had to determine was whether Jack was clinically depressed. I also wanted to figure out whether he was doing poorly in school because he was depressed or depressed because he was doing poorly in school.

In my experience, doing poorly in school usually precedes the onset of depression. But since clinical depression is easier to treat than laziness—not to mention more potentially fatal—it has to be carefully ruled out.

Even when it's the result of the poor academic performance rather than the cause, the depression may still be severe enough to require treatment. Once triggered, depression can take on a life of its own, making academic work nearly impossible and creating a vicious circle of failure leading to depression, leading to more failure. Treating the depression breaks the vicious circle and gives you the chance to apply yourself more effectively to your academic work.

But sometimes, when the workload feels overwhelming, or the shame of having screwed up is too hard to face, you may be tempted to cling to your depression and "refuse" to get better. Though genuine, at least at the onset of the episode, the depression is later put to use as an excuse for avoiding schoolwork. Only after antidepressants have failed to bring about a sustained improvement, and the psychotherapy has stalled, does the (sometimes unconscious) resistance to giving up the depression become apparent. And only then does the real work of treatment begin.

Fortunately, Jack was not clinically depressed.

"I was feeling depressed until I told my parents what was happening," he explained. "Once I made the decision to take a leave from school and come home, I felt a lot better. Now I just miss my friends."

For the rest of the initial consultation, Jack filled me in on his academic history, his life at school, and his relationship with his parents, which had been strained over the years by his poor work habits and frustrating tendency to procrastinate.

Jack had done well in school until the sixth grade. There were some symptoms suggestive of mild ADD—restlessness and daydreaming in class, distractibility and procrastination doing homework, and difficulty reading challenging books like *The Scarlet Letter*, which he started but didn't manage to finish, in ninth grade. Because of his charm and native intelligence, both his parents and his teachers had given Jack lots of encouragement and help structuring his work. As Jack put it, "I was bright enough to do well without having to kill myself."

In middle and high school, as the workload and distractions increased and the effects of puberty began to exert their influence, Jack started to perform less well. He noticed that some of the smart kids seemed to do well without doing much work, and he decided to emulate them. Still, he continued to play football in the fall, basketball in the winter, and lacrosse in the spring—all of which made him happy. His teachers gave him plenty of direction and latitude when necessary. His parents made sure nothing fell through the cracks, reminded him when his assignments were due, and pushed him as best they could to get his work done. So Jack did pretty well. He wasn't at the top of his class, but he wasn't at the bottom either.

In his senior year of high school, Jack applied early to the University of North Carolina but was rejected. After that, things went downhill. His heart went out of doing schoolwork and went instead into partying with his friends. He stayed out late and began smoking pot almost daily. He was lucky to get into the first-rate college that accepted him in April.

Jack did well his first semester in college. He had decided to turn over a new leaf after high school and mostly succeeded in doing so. During the second semester, Jack lost a little momentum but still managed to finish his freshman year with a B average.

After a great summer teaching basketball at sleep-away camp, Jack moved with three of his friends into an apartment off campus and began his sophomore year. He and his roommates were excited about living together. They agreed that, since nothing much happened in class for the first few weeks anyway, they could safely spend their time watching TV, tossing a Frisbee on the quad, playing video games, planning house parties, drinking beer, and smoking pot. After the first month, however, two of his three roommates began doing their schoolwork. Not Jack. He hung out with the one roommate who was still slacking off.

"I've always been able to learn what I need to just by going to class," he explained. "I never do any of the reading until I have to write a paper or take an exam. I seem to be able to skim the reading or find stuff I need on the Internet in order to do well."

"Once I get into my work," he continued. "I usually like it. It's just hard to get started. And if I don't really like the subject matter or the teacher, I more or less stop working altogether. That's why, even though I have a B-minus average, my grades are all over the map."

Jack explained that professors who seemed passionate about their subjects, were strict about deadlines and grades but gave as much as they demanded, brought out the best in him. Professors who were unprepared or winged it in class, seemed bored by what they were teaching or were lax in enforcing good behavior, brought out the worst in him. (Based on his grades, the number of professors Jack considered good and the number he considered bad were about equally divided.)

At the end of his sophomore year, Jack had managed to pass both semesters employing his usual m.o., although he had to take an incomplete and agree to finish three overdue assignments for that class before the start of the fall semester.

To work on his incomplete, Jack reluctantly took an office job in the city that summer instead of going away to camp. Having him at home gave Jack's parents a chance to witness his "laziness" firsthand. They couldn't help themselves: they started nagging him about going to bed and sleeping late, watching too much TV, and putting off work on his overdue papers. Despite their nagging (although he claimed *because* of their nagging), Jack never managed to complete his three assignments from the spring term before returning to school in the fall. He began his junior year already behind in his work and already demoralized.

"I couldn't get going at all this semester," he said. "Maybe I should have taken more of a break over the summer. All I did when I got back to school was watch TV and smoke pot. Two of my roommates got so pissed off they refused to hang out with me. I missed more and more classes, and fell further and further behind, until I didn't know what to do. I knew my parents would be really disappointed. I felt so hopeless and overwhelmed I couldn't get out of bed. I brought a bunch of books home over Thanksgiving, hoping to try to catch up a little bit. But I got nothing done. When I got back to school, I just collapsed."

I asked Jack why, despite his good intentions and knowing what he was supposed to do, things had gotten so out of control.

"I don't know," he answered. "Procrastination?"

When I met with Jack and his parents the following week, his father had a different answer, which he expressed with great conviction. "Jack's lazy!" he said. "Things have always come easily to Jack, so he's never learned how to work. We pushed him through high school and, now that we're not there to push him, he can't—or *won't*—do it for himself."

Naturally, Jack protested when his father made his bald assertion about Jack's laziness. He was more agreeable when his mother offered that he might have a smidgen of ADD. But privately, when we met alone again, Jack acknowledged that laziness, or at least its symptoms—procrastination, avoidance, slap-dash work, and rationalization—was a distinct possibility.

The Cure for Laziness

So now what? If laziness is the problem, what is the solution? Can laziness be cured?

The short answer is that I don't know whether laziness per se can be cured. Certainly, there is no easy formula for overcoming laziness—though it doesn't surprise me that lazy people (I include myself here) should want to find one. Fortunately, true laziness—in the sense of not *wanting* to work—is pretty rare. And although the symptoms associated with laziness—like procrastination and avoidance—are not rare, they can at least be treated if not actually cured.

The treatment for laziness is to adopt the behaviors of people who aren't lazy. People who aren't lazy function differently from people who are. Lazy people are like thoroughbred racehorses. Nonlazy people are like workhorses.

Though unduly flattering to the lazy and insulting to the nonlazy, these similes capture an essential truth. Like thoroughbreds, lazy people are very temperamental. They're finely tuned: when all the conditions are optimal, they can turn in a good performance. But if *anything* is off kilter—how much sleep they've had, how hungry they are, how quiet the room is, etc.—lazy people won't get out of the gate. And if they're not doing better than the competition after the race is underway, they're tempted to give up.

Nonlazy people are like workhorses: they get moving as soon as they're put in harness and they keep going until the day is done. They don't require perfect conditions or constant whipping and praise to do their job. They don't stop because they're tired or hungry, because there's commotion in the hallway, or they've been working all week. They do what they're supposed to do.

Your goal should be to study the habits of workhorses and become more like them.

I can tell you some general and specific methods nonlazy people use to get work done—methods you can learn and master too. But *wanting* to employ those methods won't be enough. You'll actually have to employ them, which means, ironically, that you'll have to *overcome* your laziness in order to treat it!

Six Principles for Overcoming Laziness

All the methods that help overcome laziness are based on six general principles:

1. *Treat the Treatable.*
If you *do* have a treatable disorder, get it treated. Undiagnosed or untreated, ADD, OCD, depression, or anxiety are like a backback full of bricks. They make reading and writing much more painful than they are for other people. Your laziness may be a learned response to feeling overwhelmed whenever you sit down to work. Treating these disorders will remove the backpack of bricks. You'll still have to unlearn your bad work habits. But, when you *do* sit down to work, you'll feel less overwhelmed and the work will go more easily.

2. Make work less painful.

Since lazy people find work more unpleasant than nonlazy people, it makes sense to find techniques that will make work feel less unpleasant. Some people listen to music to provide a mental lift or work in the library where they'll be inspired by other people. Others reward themselves after a couple of hours with snacks or a workout. Of course, some unpleasantness will still remain—that's what makes work *work*. But finding ways to make work less onerous will lower your resistance to doing it.

3. Know yourself.

In trying to make work less painful, it pays to know yourself. Figure out what interferes with your capacity to work and what enhances it. This is a difficult thing to do, because it requires being honest with yourself at precisely the moment when you'd most like to make excuses.

Do you thrive on competition? Find a challenging class or a demanding instructor. Do you avoid competition unless you know you can win? Convince yourself to study for the sake of knowledge and not for the grades. Tend to be a little grandiose? Be careful not to take courses over your head. Get lonely and distracted studying in your room? Go to the library. Get distracted in the library? Find a quiet study carrel. Spend too much time on YouTube or Facebook? Don't bring your earphones or log onto the net.

4. It's easier to continue work than to start it.

The greatest resistance to doing work is at its initiation. Once started, work has a way of drawing you in that makes it easier to continue. This could be considered the academic equivalent of Newton's First Law of Motion: bodies at rest remain at rest and bodies in motion remain in motion unless acted upon by an external force. (Hopefully the external force is your own motivation and not an academic dean threatening you with probation.) You want to overcome inertia and establish momentum. Let's call it the First Law of Academic Motion.

The easiest way to initiate work is to have a routine. You don't want to wake up every morning and ask yourself *Should I work?* or, worse, *Do I feel like working?*—because a high percentage of the time the answer will be no. If you've established a routine of starting work every morning at 10:00 A.M., you won't have to ask and answer the question: Should I work? You'll already be doing it.

5. Make work the first thing you do.

It's always tempting to do something pleasant before starting the "unpleasant" job of studying or writing. You'll want to check your e-mail or the news online, clean your room, eat a snack, or hang out with friends. But, once you start those other activities, they have a way of continuing for many hours (the First Law of Academic Motion). Pretty soon you've given up on the idea of work altogether.

"Getting organized" is not the same as doing work. It's another time waster. If you start an assignment or do required reading the moment you think of it, you may be less "organized," but you'll get more done. Organize yourself tonight before you go to bed so you can get down to work first thing tomorrow morning.

6. Have a goal.

Try to come up with a concrete and specific reason why you need to study what you're studying *right now*. It shouldn't be something vague—like *I want to learn for the sake of learning, my parents will be proud of me if I do well* or *I won't be able to get a job without a degree*. It should be something specific—like *I want to become an expert on Shakespearean sonnets, get into medical school, or get a job at McKinsey*. If you're studying the environmental and economic issues of global warming, imagine trying to win an argument with an oil lobbyist or with Al Gore. If you're studying the battle of Gettysburg, imagine having to explain it clearly and vividly to a class of really smart tenth graders.

I know, you're supposed to be in college to grow intellectually, to challenge your preconceptions about the world, and to become an informed citizen. And you *should* do all those things. But if you're having trouble motivating yourself to do your schoolwork right now, those lofty goals might be a bit too abstract or general. Set a concrete and specific goal that will make what you're doing seem relevant. It doesn't matter whether you actually end up pursuing the goal you've chosen for yourself. You can change your goal as you go. And it doesn't matter if you have no clue what you'd like to do once you graduate. Your goal can pertain to your undergraduate major rather than to your future career. What does matter is that your goal be as concrete and specific as you can make it and that what you're studying now is critical to its attainment.

The Virtuous Circle

The easiest and least stressful method for achieving academic success is to create a virtuous circle: you work steadily and efficiently, which makes you feel prepared, which makes classroom participation and assignments more enjoyable, which results in good grades and recognition from the professor, which leads to more enthusiasm for the material, which leads back to hard work.

If the circle doesn't begin with steady and efficient work, however, it won't end up being virtuous. If you somehow manage to get good grades without having really earned them, you won't feel motivated to work hard (you may feel motivated to "be effortlessly brilliant"—a bad thing) and you won't feel enthused about what you're studying. Worse, if you don't work steadily and efficiently, you may start a *vicious* circle—skipped classes, late assignments, poor exam results, low grades, discouragement, self-loathing, and, eventually, giving up.

It all comes back to the First Law of Academic Motion: overcoming inertia and maintaining momentum.

The Threshold Effect

As far as I know there is no such thing as the Threshold Effect in pedagogy. It's a term I made up by analogy to the Energy of Activation in chemistry because, like the First Law of Academic Motion, it sounds scientific. What it really means is that the biggest hurdle to doing work comes at the beginning of a task, when you're just getting started. Once you get over the hump and get rolling, it's much easier to continue.

The Threshold Effect applies both to the beginning of the semester when you're trying to learn new and unfamiliar material and to the beginning of an individual study session when you're trying to sit down and start your work. This is the time when the work seems the hardest and when the temptation to procrastinate is the greatest. The key, then, is to start your work immediately and not to stop until you've gotten over the threshold. Start working the first day of the term so you can get over the hump of vacation lethargy and the challenge of learning new material. And begin each individual study session as soon as possible after the class where the work was assigned so you can get over the resistance to getting started.

Once you've learned the basics of a subject, it becomes easier to acquire new information, which means the earlier you get started, the easier the rest of the term will be. And the earlier you initiate your work each day and make it beyond the Threshold Effect, the easier it is to put in the time necessary to succeed.

Make a pledge to sit down and start your work—and not stop until you're over the Threshold Effect. Once you're really rolling, *keep going*. Don't squander your momentum by taking a long break and having to overcome the Threshold Effect all over again. As the semester proceeds, your intellectual and psychological muscles will get stronger, and it will be easier and easier to overcome the Threshold Effect and persevere until your work is done.

Jack, the college junior who took a leave of absence before the end of his first semester, gave me a beautiful example of how the Threshold Effect could work for him or against him.

Before he returned to college for the spring semester, Jack and I confirmed his mother's suspicion that he did indeed have attention deficit disorder (ADD). I started him on the stimulant medication Adderall with impressive results. For the first time in his life, Jack was able to read for several hours without getting up to surf the net or get a snack. He could absorb what he was reading without having to reread every page. And he was able to structure essays in his mind without having to waste time "getting organized." In short, Jack was able to focus on his academic work in a way that allowed him to fulfill his potential.

By reducing distractibility, the stimulant medication lowered Jack's threshold to starting and continuing work. But there was a hitch. It took thirty minutes for the medication to get into his system and take effect. What Jack did during that thirty-minute window was critical. If he began his schoolwork during that half-hour interval (even though his attention was not yet 100 percent), he would glide effortlessly into a productive day of studying and writing. But, if he checked sports scores online instead, he would continue to surf the Web with rapt attention for the many hours.

The lesson? Strike while the iron is hot. Do your academic work before doing anything else.

SPECIFIC METHODS FOR IMPROVING ACADEMIC PERFORMANCE

Here are some specific methods that have proven helpful for other people and may be helpful for you.

Take a Summer Course

This may be my best piece of academic advice: Take an introductory level college course during your summer vacation. Choose a college near your home, not the college you will be attending in the fall. You can do this the summer before starting college or before your sophomore year. Taking it before you start college has two advantages: 1.

It prepares you to cope with the academic demands of college *before* you've had a chance to flounder. It's preventive rather than remedial. 2. It helps to polish off some of the academic rust caused by the corrosive effect of senioritis and helps you to gain academic momentum. Taking a course during sophomore summer is helpful in regaining confidence if you've done less well than you should have freshman year.

Another good time to take a summer course is after a year or semester abroad. Since most study-abroad courses depend less on rigorous academic work and more on "experiential learning" (often interpreted as partying in Paris or imbibing in England), many students return to school in the fall not having done any serious schoolwork for half a year. They find it hard to buckle down at the very time their grades count the most—their senior year. Taking a course during the intervening summer will help get you back in shape for the final push.

The best offering to choose for your summer prep is an "Introduction to" course in a subject you're generally good at but that will not likely be your major. A course you're interested in that will fulfill a distribution requirement is ideal. Summer courses are usually briefer and more intense than fall and spring semester courses, but are also somewhat less academically rigorous, which makes them easier to ace. Because you can't usually transfer the letter grade to your transcript—you generally get only pass/fail credit—there is also less anxiety and pressure in taking a course at a different college. You should, however, arrange transfer credit at your own college in advance so that you can get something other than a positive experience out of taking your summer course. Taking the course for credit is motivating and having an extra credit in hand will allow you to drop a course during the regular year if you're failing or get overwhelmed.

Some institutions won't give credit for courses taken at other colleges prior to your freshman year. If this is the case at your college, check with the first-year dean to see if an exemption can be made. You may need to take your summer "prep" course at the college you will be attending in the fall to get credit. Of course, this means leaving home earlier than anticipated, but it also gives you a head start on adjusting to your new school.

The idea behind this exercise is to ace a single course by doing all the work that's required from beginning to end. Once you've figured out how to master *this* college course, you will understand what it takes to master *any* college course. And once you've tasted what it's like to be totally on top of your work—to feel confident in your ability to work effectively, excited by what you're studying, able to participate in classroom discussion instead of hoping the professor won't call on you, and be at the upper end of the bell curve instead of in the middle—you will never want to go back to being a slacker again.

You can combine your summer course with part-time work but *not* with any other academic pursuits. Because it's only one course, you should be able to apply enough discipline to accomplish all the basics and go that extra mile to excel without feeling too stressed. And it's important that you devote yourself to doing so, because succeeding now will make it much harder to *not* succeed later on. Once you've been an academic standout, it's hard to go back to being a mediocrity.

Think of this course as preseason in the same way college athletes do when they show up to campus early to prepare for the football or field hockey season. Don't procrastinate or use the excuse that it's your summer vacation. There ought to be plenty of time for other part-time work and socializing with friends. Don't stay up late drinking before your classes. Do all your work before going out. Take this exercise seriously and you'll learn how to set priorities and fit things into your schedule. College will become surprisingly manageable. And you'll have a set of skills that will help you throughout your life.

Choose Courses Wisely

1. Once you're in school, try to choose courses that are neither too difficult nor too easy. Avoid being grandiose: Don't conclude that, because you're intending to apply to medical school, you should be smart enough to take all the most advanced science courses or com-

plete all the requirements in the first year. (Many premed students, for example, take organic chemistry over the summer when they can devote more time to it.)

Take courses you can do well in and spread out the hard ones over several terms. Don't choose courses that are so easy that you're likely to get bored: it will only encourage you to devalue the subject matter and cultivate grandiosity and poor work habits. But don't choose courses that are so hard that you'll get discouraged and give up your academic goals.

And don't kid yourself that this will be the course where you finally start to do all the work and live up to your potential. Be honest with yourself about your actual odds of success. If you've never worked to capacity before, don't assume you're going to do so now.

2. Diversify your portfolio. Choose courses that will give variety to your classroom experience (seminars, labs, lectures), study methods (reading, problem sets), and evaluation techniques (essays, exams, research projects, class participation). Take courses that differ in subject matter, workload, and difficulty. Just for fun, take an easy course that interests you.

3. *Don't* diversify your portfolio. If you hate writing papers and prefer to cram for exams, take courses that are graded entirely on the midterm and final exams—generally large lecture courses. If studying for exams gives you ulcers, but handing in regular assignments, writing papers, and participating in classroom discussions helps you keep up with your work, take classes that downplay exams—generally small seminar courses.

4. Find professors who are great teachers and fair markers. Taking a subject you're less interested in with an outstanding teacher is usually more rewarding, in every sense, than taking a beloved subject with a lousy teacher.

Use student evaluations and word of mouth to do your research. But use multiple sources and take any single evaluation with a grain of salt.

5. If you like to have your hand held or need mentoring, choose courses where the professor knows your name and cares about how you do. If you prefer to fly under the radar, take large lecture courses where you can chug along in relative obscurity.

6. Register for an extra course during the shopping period in case you have to drop a course later. If the registrar's computer limits the number of courses you can register for, get the instructor's permission to enroll in her course and finalize your course registration after you've decided what courses you want to retain. This avoids scrambling about trying to find a suitable course from those that still have open enrollment, and it keeps you from falling behind by several weeks and having to play catch-up.

7. Care about good grades. If you're able to get honors, don't settle for a pass. Getting good grades is motivating. Starting off your freshman year with good grades will make school more fun and encourage you to want to continue putting in the effort to succeed. Yes, there is something noble about pursuing knowledge for its own sake—consequences be damned. But there is nothing ignoble or anti-intellectual about choosing courses that will permit you to get good grades. Doing poorly, especially at the beginning of your college career, is dispiriting. Although most students do better in their junior and senior years, once they get the hang of course selection and are able to concentrate on one or two areas of specialization, starting strong is a huge leg up.

Simplify

Whatever your supposed level of sophistication, start your study of a subject *at least* one level below where you think you are. No one has ever suffered from brushing up on the basics or reviewing first principles before moving on to more challenging material. Get out your old elementary textbook on the subject. And don't just read it over, *master* the material—it ought to be easier and faster the second time around. Bring the level of complexity down to the point where you can grasp the central concepts and employ them to solve problems or decipher novel situations. Only then should you ratchet up the level of complexity. Do this especially if you've been away from the subject for a while, such as after a summer break, study abroad, or leave of absence.

Mastering the basics before going on to the current material will be time well spent. Most professors devote a fair proportion of their tests to the basics, even in the upper levels. And for good reason—because you can't really understand the complex stuff unless you thoroughly understand the simple stuff. Even if *all* you manage to learn is the basics, there's still a pretty good chance you'll pass the course.

Mastering or remastering the basics will make you adept in the subject. By uncovering unexpected gaps in your existing knowledge, you'll build confidence for the new. And, by being fluent in your understanding of the first principles, you'll be more creative and more able to make connections you might not otherwise have seen. Brilliant scientists and scholars are brilliant *because* they're able to see complex problems simply, often by reasoning from first principles.

Create a Routine and Stick to It

It's very hard to acquire discipline by applying willpower. The best way to acquire discipline is by imposing structure. If you want to sharpen your skills and become a better student, try to establish and follow a daily and weekly routine. Do the same thing, at the same time, for the same duration, in the same location, on the same day every week. It's hard to do this as a college student. But, remember, you're trying to turn over a new leaf and build new skills. When you're setting up your routine, start out being as rigorous as possible. This applies as much to when you eat, sleep, and exercise as to when you attend classes, study, and work on assignments.

If you're religious about following your schedule, you will find that getting everything done will become easier and easier. Your stamina, perseverance, and proficiency will increase. And your discipline will become a wonder, even to you. In time, you'll be able to introduce some flexibility into your routine without sacrificing productivity or self-discipline.

Keep a Sharp Boundary Between Work and Play

On Sundays I love to get up late, read the *New York Times* over a leisurely cup of coffee, stay in my pajamas until 11:00 A.M., and, if I can, avoid shaving until Monday. If I started weekday mornings like that, however, I'd never get anything accomplished.

As a corollary to establishing and sticking to a routine, and making work the first activity you do, there is the principle of separating work from play. You're entitled to some downtime. The trick is to confine your downtime to weekends, the occasional evening (except when even your weekends and evenings are needed for work), and to reserve your weekdays and most evenings for work.

I had a patient who made sure his classes were scheduled around noon so he could get up at 9:00 A.M. and have a relaxed morning beforehand. He'd make breakfast for half an hour after getting up, watch a show on ESPN for an hour, and then go online for an hour to catch up on sports scores or play a video game. He assumed this strategy would be better than his prior one of getting out of bed at 11:00 A.M. and gobbling down a late breakfast before running to his noon class where he'd arrive disorganized and frazzled.

The only problem with his new relaxed approach was that he got so caught up in relaxing that he couldn't bring himself to spoil it by going to his noon class at all—or doing his work before or after. If he *did* manage to get to his noon class, he felt he needed a bit of a breather afterward (a little play mingled in with his work), so he'd have a leisurely lunch, a nap, and then more video games. Whatever work he did he started after supper—but by then he was generally "tired," so little or nothing was accomplished.

My point in relating this anecdote is to encourage you to keep the weekends and the occasional evening for play and to devote your days to schoolwork. If you *do* succumb to temptation and end up playing during your work time, cleanse your palette by taking a walk or working out so that your mind is clear when you finally start your work.

Interposing a physical activity between the mental activities of playing video games or surfing the net and doing schoolwork sharpens the boundary between play and work. Since play is generally more fun, it's important to keep that boundary sharp to prevent it from encroaching on your work.

Keep Focused on the Task at Hand

Focus on the present moment, not on the past or future. If you're supposed to be studying, don't think about the troubling conversation you had with your boyfriend or the test you have tomorrow morning. It's hard not to worry about those things, but doing so is a distraction from your present task. Indeed, if you permit yourself to worry about the past and future, you may be *trying* to avoid the task at hand. Don't do it.

Worrying about the past and future, which you can't control, prevents you from focusing on the present, which you can. Save thoughts about the past and future for your spare time, when doing so won't interfere with the present and may even be useful.

Focus on the *task*, not the *result*. Of course you should want to do well, but, if you focus on the result (getting an A) instead of on the task (trying to improve your knowledge and skills), you'll shift your focus from something you *can* control to something you *can't*. You may want to get an A on an essay, but you can't really control that. You can only control how skillfully you research and write your paper. Not surprisingly, when you focus on the task rather than the result, you often end up with a result you can be proud of.

Manage Expectations

Be realistic about how much work you're likely to do. Don't take on more than you can handle. You have four years to complete your undergraduate education (although many students take five or more years). You don't have to do everything in the first couple of years. Reserve some of the challenges for when you're in your junior and senior years and better able to choose and manage your courses.

To that end:

1. Don't be grandiose: Don't skip the introductory courses just because you've taken the AP exam in the subject. College-level courses are usually more rigorous than the equivalent AP courses. In any case, it doesn't hurt to review the material one more time, give yourself a firm foundation for the more advanced courses, and, as a result, get a good grade (no small thing).

2. Don't be perfectionistic: You may be brilliant. Nevertheless, it's unlikely you're going to blow away your professor with your undergraduate work. Better to do a creditable job and get that economics paper done than to do a brilliant job and turn it in late or never. The problem gets worse once you've missed a deadline, because then the pressure to redeem yourself gets more intense. Feeling the need to produce something spectacular lowers the chance you'll get around to producing anything at all. Remember: the perfect is the enemy of the good.

3. Don't be overly sensitive to criticism: you are in college to learn. Expect criticism and don't take it personally. Whatever you do, don't give up. Many a great writer, scientist, artist, physician, etc. stumbled at the beginning of her training. And too many potentially successful writers, scientists, artists, doctors, etc. gave up prematurely because some putative authority told them they didn't have what it takes. Don't be discouraged if not all your grades are as high as you would like. Most people get a few Cs during their college careers. Your only goal should be to make the effort to do well.

4. Don't be overly competitive: everyone's coursework is different. Your goal should be to do as well as *you* can, not to be the best. If you happen to be taking a program you love, for which you have great ap-

titude, you may end up being the best. But that will be a fortunate by-product of your enthusiasm and hard work, not a direct goal.

HOW TO COPE WITH A HEAVY READING LOAD— AND STAY AWAKE WHILE DOING SO

Pleasure Reading Versus Academic Reading

Let me begin with an observation: If you picked up *Anna Karenina* to read at the beach over the summer (not a likely scenario, I know, but stay with me on this), you would probably be able to read it, without putting it down, from the moment you woke up in the morning to the moment you fell asleep at night. And (unless the sun and waves got to you) you wouldn't fall asleep because the book was making you drowsy, but only because you'd been awake until 2 A.M. the night before trying to finish it.

If you were assigned five chapters of *Anna Karenina* by your comp lit professor, however, there's a good chance you'd be nodding off after a couple of pages. (And that's Tolstoy. Now picture yourself trying to stay awake through five chapters of your cultural anthropology text-book.) The reason that it's harder to get through reading you've been assigned than through reading you've picked up for your own plea-sure is that there's no anxiety associated with reading for pleasure. When you're reading something you've been assigned, you feel you have to learn every fact, theme, and argument—and that can make the book a slog.

How do you cope with an overwhelming reading load? The best way would be to turn assigned reading into pleasure reading by imag-ining you were reading at the beach. Since that isn't always (in fact, rarely) possible, another approach is to alternate your reading of an assigned text between pleasure reading and academic reading.

During the pleasure reading phase, you'd read as you would at the beach, enjoying the story or the argument without worrying unduly about remembering the facts. You'd allow yourself to become im-mersed in the narrative stream, absorbing the overarching themes and ideas of the book holistically without getting hung up on the details.

After a suitable period of time (perhaps at the end of a section), you'd stop pleasure reading and switch to academic reading. You'd make notes, set down important facts, and record your own ideas and impressions for later use.

If your pleasure reading is absorbing enough, and your academic breaks frequent enough, you ought to be able to do your note taking from memory. Your academic reading will not detract from your pleasure reading and you'll be able to get into a satisfying and productive groove.

Not having to make the exhausting and distracting effort of keeping the facts straight in your head while you're reading for pleasure might—*might*—make it possible for you to absorb the important themes and overarching ideas of the book organically, which is what good authors intend. The notes you take of the facts and of your own insights and ideas during the academic breaks will permit you to study or write essays later, without having to reread the entire text.

Selective Reading

Another way to cope with an overwhelming reading load is by cheating or, as most undergraduates prefer to think of it, "reading selectively."

If you're going to cheat, however, cheat intelligently. Figure out what's important to read and read it carefully. Since the important stuff is usually introduced at the beginning, developed in the middle, and summarized at the end, the smartest way to cut corners is by reading the beginning and the end of a passage, skipping the middle.

So, if you're overwhelmed and unable to read everything you've been assigned, you can at least try to read 1. the introduction and the first and last chapters of a book, 2. the first and last paragraphs of a chapter, and 3. the first and last sentences of a paragraph. (I first heard about this method of "selective reading" from a successful public interest attorney with ADD who'd used it to get through law school.)

It would be hard to read most introductory textbooks, overview articles, scientific and technical treatises, or literary works this way. And it would be hard to follow a well-reasoned argument or mathematical proof this way. But, for secondary sources (such as critiques and interpretations of a literary text) and books and articles in the social sciences and humanities, this method of "selective reading" might just do the trick in a pinch. It's certainly better than doing no reading at all.

For readings that contain really complicated arguments, for texts where the facts are important (history, physics, Latin), and for ideas that are novel, or poorly expressed, create notes that make the arguments, facts, and ideas clear to you. You will become engaged by the intellectual challenge of trying to summarize the text and gratified by having untied the intellectual knots—and that too will make the reading less of a slog.

If you hate reading, or are hobbled by ADD or some other problem that makes reading a chore, take good lecture notes and study from them. Failing that, try to acquire good lecture notes from willing classmates or search for relevant course material online. Sometimes the lectures and syllabi from the same course at another college are better organized and more comprehensible. In a pinch, there are always CliffsNotes.

Of course, you *could* try to stay awake when you're reading by drinking cup after cup of coffee or popping someone else's Ritalin or Adderall. But, since your daytime drowsiness is psychological (boredom and avoidance), not physiological (sleep deprivation), it's unlikely to work. What caffeine and stimulants *will* do, however, is give you insomnia that night. Then your drowsiness next day will be both psychological *and* physiological.

Optimize Work Conditions

1. Find a good place to study where you won't be distracted, restless, or bored. For many people the library helps overcome the

loneliness and boredom that accompanies studying. It provides just the right amount of stimulation, camaraderie, and encouragement to keep you from falling asleep or looking for distractions.

2. Some people like to reduce distractions by finding a room that is dead silent. Others like to reduce distractions by using quiet music as white noise. What you shouldn't do is stay online on the net while you're using your computer to study or write papers. Turn off your mobile phone and don't text, IM, e-mail, or read breaking news bulletins. While you're at it, turn off the TV.

By the way, it's not critical to Tweet about your every activity, keep your Facebook profile current, create albums of yourself drunk at costume parties, poke each of your thousand "friends," or write daily messages on their walls. You could actually decide to do your schoolwork instead.

3. Working with a study partner may help you to stay motivated. Teaching each other will help you to learn the material and obligate you to keep up your end of the bargain.

Even if you don't have a study partner or partners, at least avoid the company of people who will lead you astray. Watch out for cynics, know-it-alls, braggarts, liars, downers, online gamers, and naive idealists who think that doing something in college to better mankind takes precedence over bettering yourself.

Be wary of people who make you feel inadequate. If *you* are one of those people (and, at one or another time, we all are), examine why you're behaving this way. The reason is usually obvious—you're unhappy and want to make yourself feel better at the expense of those who seem happy. Remember, it's more satisfying to remedy a problem than to drag others down with you.

4. Make it a practice *not* to end your homework at its natural endpoint. End your homework somewhere *after* the beginning of the next section. For example, don't stop studying at the end of a chapter, stop studying after the beginning of the *next* chapter. Don't stop writ-

ing an essay at the end of one section; end it a paragraph or two into the next section.

By ending your work well into the next task, you will lower the Threshold Effect of resuming that task when you next pick it up. If you take a break prematurely—especially if the break is a "legitimate" one (like eating lunch, doing laundry, exercising, etc.)—you will find it easier to *avoid* getting back to work later. And, as we all know, avoidance has a way of feeding on itself.

5. Finally, as I mentioned earlier, strike while the iron is hot. Perform tasks immediately. Don't spend time creating a framework for starting things. Start them. It's easier to initiate activities while they're still fresh in your mind than to do so after they've begun to degrade. Letting things pile up makes it more likely you'll procrastinate or avoid doing them altogether.

This applies to small things as well as big and to activities of daily living as well as schoolwork. If you dirty a dish, for example, wash it right away—don't just put it in the sink. If you get an idea for an essay, write it down and start writing the essay—don't just try to keep it in the back of your mind. Putting off doing the little things causes them to build up into big things. Letting the dishes pile up results in an hour of wasted time trying to scrape them clean when you finally get around to doing them. Failing to record or act upon an idea that's occurred to you while reading or walking between classes usually results in forgetting the idea altogether.

Take One Day at a Time

Taking one day at a time—a motto made popular by Alcoholics Anonymous—is a good tactic for dealing with procrastination. Actually, in AA, they break it down further to one hour or one minute at a time—a mantra that allows people to resist relapse moment by moment without the pressure of "changing for good." The problem with procrastination is that, when you give in to it once, you're tempted to keep giving in to it over and over again until you hit rock bottom. We all do it: *I got a late start this morning; the day is wasted anyway; there's no point in starting now; I'll start my assignment tomorrow.*

Wouldn't it be great if there were a twelve-step program for procrastinators? Call it PA. I think it would be helpful beyond "one day at a time." Twelve-step programs offer tolerant, nonjudgmental support and fellowship for people struggling with overwhelming temptation (in the case of procrastinators, the temptation to avoid stressful or tedious work). They destigmatize the behavior they're confronting, which increases the likelihood that procrastinators will actually confront their problems. And they provide concrete steps for making needed changes. Though forgiving, these programs aspire to rigorous honesty. While acknowledging human frailty, they insist on integrity, commitment, and responsibility (first to yourself, then to others.) And, though optimistic, they accept the prospect of life-long effort.

PA would give procrastinators the nonjudgmental support they need to confront their addiction to avoidance. There ought to be a chapter on every college campus.

In any case, the advantage of taking one day at a time (or, better still, one hour at a time) is, if you procrastinate at nine o'clock, you don't have to waste the rest of the day. You can start at ten o'clock. It's less daunting to commit to working for an hour at a time than for a whole day or a whole semester. If you commit to doing your work for *this* hour, you can recommit *next* hour when it becomes this hour. You're less likely to balk at doing your work if you don't have to commit to two hours from the get-go.

THE SPECIAL PROBLEMS OF THE GIFTED AND LAZY

Accepting the Need to Work

Over the years, I've treated quite a number of students who seem to embody a perfect storm of self-defeating character traits—perfectionism, grandiosity, avoidance, laziness, and paralyzing (though un-conscious) fear of disappointing their parents and teachers. I think a lot of you will recognize yourselves in what I'm about to describe. (I would have recognized myself in this description when I was in college.)

If you're gifted and lazy, you were probably precociously verbal as a child, which, instead of making you diligent and productive, made you a bit lazy and spoiled. You regard yourself as special and are often treated as such by your teachers and parents (and even by your parents' friends).

Unfortunately, being special makes struggling with difficult course material or persevering with mundane assignments seem unfair, if not downright insulting. Teachers love you "not wisely but too well," rewarding bursts of brilliance more than dogged determination. On the rare occasion you are criticized by your teachers, you feel wounded and angry and tempted to give up. You're impatient with tedious labor and disdainful of conventional ideas, both of which you see as mediocre. For you mediocrity is worse than failure.

And failure is inevitable. In college, the material gets too challenging and the workload too heavy to be mastered without some slogging.

If you're not honest with yourself about the need to work, your bad habits will be reinforced. Having failed to win recognition by excelling academically, you will turn your efforts towards other sources of acclaim—some good, some not so good. The good ones—like writing for a student publication, volunteering in the community, managing an organization, or performing in plays, musicals, and improvisation groups, etc.—can instill a work ethic, forge lifelong friendships, and launch a career. The not so good ones—like becoming a campus radical, a druggie, or an eccentric—can lead to isolation, despair, and marginalization.

But, if you are honest with yourself about the need to work, a taste of failure will reform your character. You'll overcome your aversion to work and begin to earn real accolades through real effort. If you're lucky, you'll be taken under the wing of an alert and responsible professor who, by a skillful combination of encouragement and toughness, will get you to perform. But even if you have to do it on your own—*especially* if you have to do it on your own—you *will* perform. Why? Because you're not just gifted and lazy, you're ambitious as well.

Avoiding Becoming a Phony

There is a specific danger that confronts you if you're gifted and lazy and have lost your self-confidence because of academic floundering. You may want to regain your confidence, or at least the *appearance* of having regained your confidence, by adopting a persona that seems immune to the embarrassment of having done poorly in college. A persona is a fake self—an anemic version of your true self—not merely a facade. It's not the shell covering and protecting a bruised personality; it's the alien kernel that has come to fill the shell where your personality used to be. Just as a zombie is the soulless version of a living person, a persona is the pureed version of a healthy personality. If you used to be friendly and outgoing, you suddenly become sullen and antagonistic. If you were once happy and energetic, you're now morose and sickly. The problem—and the danger—is that your persona will feel real to you. You'll come to believe that the sullen, antagonistic, morose, and sickly *persona* you now are is your true self and that the friendly, outgoing, happy, and energetic *person* you used to be was a false self—and that it's gone forever.

But, if your false self now seems true and your true self now seems false, how do you know whether you've developed a zombielike persona or simply have a personality that sucks? It's hard to sort out because you created your persona for an important purpose—to conceal feelings of shame and defeat not just from the world but from yourself. Your persona helped you to regain a feeling of control over your life at a time when you felt out of control—when you felt overwhelmed and defeated.

Luckily, there is an infallible sign that the persona you think is the real you is, in truth, merely an unhealthy facsimile: you feel unhappy.

You feel there's a hole where your heart used to be. You feel vaguely ashamed and fraudulent. Even though you don't necessarily remember when the change occurred, you feel uncomfortable with the person you've turned into. Your resilience and spontaneity are shot. You feel brittle. You feel your promise has been unfulfilled. Mostly you feel that a vital part of yourself—something that once made you feel lovable and special—has been crushed.

Aaron was the son of two high school English teachers. As a child, he was not only physically beautiful but unusually charming and articulate as well. He had read *War and Peace* by the time he was in sixth grade and was fluent in French by the end of the eighth. Although he didn't work hard, his teachers admired his brilliance and rewarded him with high marks.

In the ninth grade, however, Aaron began to run into trouble at school. For his science project that year, he had set himself the task of describing the big bang theory and star formation. Having chosen a topic that was over his head and refusing to get help from his science teacher, Aaron never completed the project. He got his first ever C. Unfortunately, it was not his last.

That first C changed his life. Humiliated by his poor showing on the science project and unaccustomed to hard work, Aaron decided to adopt the persona of an intellectual—a critic of conventional ideas and lifestyles who followed his own curriculum, learned only what interested him, and displayed haughty disdain for humdrum ideas and people. In short, he became a dilettante and minor eccentric—a source of amusement to his friends but puzzlement to his parents and teachers who knew he was capable of much more.

Aaron managed to graduate high school and get into a small college in New England. But, once there, he shed what remained of his healthy personality and entered fully into his eccentric persona. He skipped classes, wrote rambling essays on idiosyncratic topics different from the ones assigned by his professors, and embarrassed himself by submitting contrarian articles to the student newspaper. Aaron walked around campus in the dead of winter without a coat and added heavy drinking to his catalog of eccentricities.

When I first met with Aaron, nearly a decade after his graduation from college, he was stuck in a low-paying job as a researcher for a literary magazine, was drinking too much, angry at the world, and clinically depressed. It took him only a few weeks on medication to get over his depression but more than a year in psychotherapy to recognize that his persona had been self-made in order to cope with his academic self-doubt. Once he understood its origins, Aaron began to renounce his self-destructive persona and take the chance of letting his true personality show through. He never quite made up the ground he had lost beginning in high school, nor did he completely relinquish his persona. But with time Aaron was able to get a better job, curb his drinking, and get married.

Like many other psychological reactions to shame and disappointment, persona formation follows well-worn pathways: You might become a *charmer*, who substitutes articulateness and charisma for performance. You might become a *rebel*, who embraces the counterculture because you're afraid to risk drowning in the mainstream. You might become an *artist*, who sacrifices worldly success for creative self-expression. You might become a *giver*, who sacrifices your own ambitions to help the downtrodden. You might become a *victim*, who blames society for your alienation and failure. Or you might become an *intellectual*, like Aaron, who consoles himself with intellectual posturing instead of striving for academic distinction.

Many personas are modeled on romantic heroes and antiheroes from books, movies, and television. The characters change from generation to generation. But what they all have in common is that they're beautiful losers, at odds with their parents, their peers, and their culture.

After a while, both from repression and the passage of time, you may forget how and why you adopted your persona. It becomes second nature, an intrinsic part of your self-image—and you begin to believe that you can never change it. You believe you've always been a charmer, a rebel, an artist, a giver, a victim, or an intellectual. More accurately, you come to believe that the charmer, rebel, artist, giver, victim, or intellectual is *all* you are.

But this isn't true. You *are* more than your persona. There *is* a real you at the heart of the beast. And it can be recovered. You *can* give up your persona and rediscover your innate personality.

How? There are two steps. First, you have to be honest with yourself. You have to remember that you constructed your persona to deal with a forgotten humiliation earlier in your life—that it isn't innate and it isn't the totality of who you are. Second, you have to be courageous. You have to be willing to renounce the melancholy comfort of your persona. You have to take the risk and do the work of leaving the false safety of your persona behind. You have to give expression to your innate personality.

You may be able to reconnect with your healthy personality on your own. But, more than likely, you'll need the objectivity, encouragement, and structure that good psychotherapy can provide.

Better than trying to deal with these maladaptive personas later in adulthood, however, is to confront them close to their inception, in college or even before, when the humiliations are still fresh and you have not yet gone too far off track. Better than therapy, in other words, is therapeutic reality—the success that comes from effort and the happiness that comes from success. Better to prevent persona formation by courageous expression of your true self and by fulfillment of your true potential during your school days than having to treat it later on in psychotherapy. But treating it later on is better than treating it not at all and continuing to live a self hollowed out at its core.

If you're one of the gifted and lazy, you can avoid developing a persona and get back on track by focusing on your studies, conferring with your professors, and embracing, rather than fighting, your work.

What to Do When You Don't Turn Over a New Leaf

At the beginning of the chapter, I told you that my suggestions on how to turn over a new leaf might not work. I'll tell you a brief story about my sessions with George and you'll see why doing what you know you're *supposed* to do can be so difficult.

George had taken a medical leave when he came to see me half-way through the fall semester of his junior year. At twenty-three, George should have been a senior but had taken so many incompletes that he was almost a year behind.

George was ambivalent about seeing me.

"My parents are worried about how I'm doing in school. They're afraid I'll end up like my uncle who's forty-three years old and never held a steady job."

"Are *you* worried?" I asked him, after having reviewed his record of academic underperformance going right back to the beginning of high school.

"Not really," he told me breezily. "I know what I have to do to succeed. I just have to actually *do* it."

"I'm sure you're right," I agreed. "Everyone pretty much knows what they have to do to succeed in college: attend class, keep up with the work, start assignments early. The problem is actually doing it. Do you have any idea why you don't do what you know you're supposed to do?"

"I don't know. All I know is that when I sit down to start a paper I end up spending three hours looking up sports news on the Web first. Sometimes I never get around to doing the paper."

George planned to return to college for the spring term, which was only a few weeks away. During our limited time, we tried to explore why he wasn't doing what he knew he was supposed to do.

I asked George whether he was using the Internet as a distraction because he was anxious about starting his work or because, as he thought, it just interested him to keep up with developments in professional sports. He wasn't sure. He wasn't *aware* of feeling anxious, but anxiety was not a feeling he had much familiarity with, so he couldn't rule it out. Luckily George did have enough self-awareness to try to make allowances for his Internet habit: instead of starting papers at 9:00 P.M. the night before they were due, as had been his custom, he now started them at 6:00 P.M. to allow for three hours of net surfing.

Once George started writing a paper, however, he really got into it. He was often intellectually fascinated by the subject matter but, because of the late start, couldn't do it justice. George also had a tendency to wander off topic into areas that interested him but weren't what the professor had asked the class to address. He spent too much of his limited time trying to prove he was original instead of getting the job done properly. With liberal professors this strategy sometimes paid off and he got a good grade; with strict professors it didn't. As a result, George's grades were all over the place: He had Bs in some courses and incompletes or Ds in others.

The other interesting thing about George was that he worked hard (for him) at internships that might lead to jobs after college. He worked reasonably hard at a paralegal job he'd had one summer and was working reasonably hard at a brokerage job he had during his current leave from school. In other words, George was capable of applying himself when the subject matter in school or at work engaged him. And he was better at applying himself consistently when he was in a structured, adult, work environment.

This led me to make a suggestion. "Why don't you treat school as if it were a job," I said. "Imagine you're not a twenty-three-year-old college student anymore. Imagine you're a twenty-nine-year-old adult who has returned to college as a mature student to get your degree—not because you're *supposed* to go to college, or because your parents want you to, but because you *want* to. You'd be doing it for *yourself*."

I continued. "You'd get up early every morning and go to the library or class as if it were a job. You'd attend every class, start every assignment on time, and do what you were asked by the professor—because you're an adult and that's what adults with jobs do."

"I've actually thought of that," George said. "I've imagined living in an apartment with a girlfriend, sitting down at my desk with a glass of wine, and doing my work."

(The glass of wine wasn't what I had in mind, and the girlfriend didn't yet exist, but I could see what George was aiming for in his fantasy—coziness, stability, and maturity—and I could see how that might help him to do his work.)

By our next appointment, however, George had reconsidered pretending to be an adult and found the idea wanting. "I don't think it's going to work," he said. "Because I've often planned to turn over a new leaf when I started a new semester. Invariably my good intentions fizzled out."

We explored the history of what happened to his good intentions at the beginning of the term. One of two things would take place, George explained: either he would spend the first few weeks catching up with his friends, socializing instead of doing his work—which would put him in catch-up mode—or he would start strong and then lose momentum. Because of the longer time *not seeing his friends*, the problem of socializing instead of doing work was worse after the summer than the winter break. Likewise, because of the longer time *not doing schoolwork*, the problem with fizzling out after a brief flurry of activity was also worse after the summer break.

"It takes me a month or so to get up the endurance to sit down and do work after the summer break," George explained. "Even half an hour of work seems like a lot, and I feel like I need—and deserve—a break."

After a few weeks, George returned to school for the next semester. I didn't feel confident that we had managed to make much headway in helping him with his inconsistent work habits.

> I suggested that he consult the study center at his college right
> away when got back.
> "I don't think I need to do that," George demurred. "I know
> what I have to do. And I think this time I'll succeed in turning
> over a new leaf."
> Needless to say, he didn't.

Why is turning over a new leaf in school so difficult? The answer
is obvious: because taking a break from schoolwork is so easy and because resuming work *after* a break is so hard.

Here's what you should do when you're unable to turn over a new
leaf on your own: GET HELP!

Don't try to tough it out. Don't lie to yourself, like George did,
that you'll be able to do it on your own, when your past history proves
otherwise. Don't flatter yourself that you're above getting help because you're too smart. Don't tell yourself you don't deserve to get
help because you haven't done any work. Don't resign yourself to the
idea that you're beyond asking for help because you're too lazy. Don't
bury your head in the sand and hope the problem will go away. GET
HELP!

Here are three places to start:

The Academic Skills Center   Most universities and colleges offer concrete suggestions on how to participate in the classroom effectively,
study various kinds of material, do research, write papers, and take
exams. These suggestions and guidelines can often be researched on
their Web sites. The McGraw Center at Princeton University has an
especially good one, but you should check out a few of them at different colleges. They're all a little different, and you could pick up a
new idea from each that might be helpful.

Checking online, however, is not enough. You should go in person
to the academic skills center at your college.

All colleges have first-year and departmental advising, student course evaluation guides, academic skills centers, learning resources, offices of disability, student counseling services, assistance

for student-athletes, writing centers, and tutors. There must be a reason why they have these programs. It can't be because academic challenges in college are rare or unique to you. And it can't be because everyone graduates from high school knowing everything there is to know about how to study, write papers, or take exams. It must be because the transition from high school to college is tough. There is no shame in availing yourself of the expertise that colleges have accumulated over many decades. The only shame would be in not doing everything you can to improve your chances of thriving.

Professors and Deans   No doubt some of you will regard the suggestion to consult with your professors and deans as unrealistic. They don't know me from Adam, I hear you thinking. And, even if they did, they have more important things to deal with than my problems anyway.

I understand why you're skeptical. I understand why you'd question whether your professors care about you or have any interest in whether or not you succeed: they're busy, they're important, and some of them *do* seem to be remote, lazy, or indifferent. But the truth is that most faculty members, including some of those who appear busy or indifferent, have had considerable experience dealing with students' academic difficulties and will want to help you. Indeed, they will feel gratified that you've turned to them for help rather than trying to go it alone.

Perhaps you're embarrassed to ask your professors for help because you brought your problems on yourself. You've skipped classes, missed deadlines, and failed to turn in assignments. You're sure your instructor will be unsympathetic—sucks to be you, he'll say. And maybe you think that's the reaction you deserve. Maybe you're gifted and lazy but, on the evidence, you figure your professor will regard you as more lazy than gifted.

Take a chance. Meet with the professor. Many academics have been gifted and lazy too in their time. They may relate to you. In any case, you have nothing to lose. Your instructors will be more likely to work with you to turn things around if you've taken the initiative to approach them than if you've simply blown them off.

If your professor *does* agree to help you, don't repay her goodwill by trying to manipulate her. Don't devalue her because she's been kind-hearted enough to give you the benefit of the doubt and cut you some slack. If you betray her trust, if you work less hard for her than for your professors who are tough, you will make it harder on your fellow students in the future. The faculty will become more skeptical and rigid—and your prejudices about their indifference will eventually become true.

After you've spoken to your instructors, talk to your dean. The dean of students and the various first-year and upper-class deans have a special interest in helping you to succeed and graduate. This is partly because they take their jobs seriously and partly because a high graduation rate helps maintain the school's reputation and standing in the rankings. Most deans have become deans not because they hate teaching but because they like helping students and their families deal with problems.

Deans are experienced in dealing with the academic, medical, substance abuse, and other problems common in your age group. They can help you deal with administrative issues, like getting extra time on assignments and taking leaves. They can help you access resources, like tutoring services and substance-abuse programs. They can approach your instructors on your behalf or advise you on how to do so. They can act as a bridge between you and your parents and the school.

Most faculty and deans, however, will not reach out to you. You will have to reach out to them. You will hear this advice many times during college orientation. Believe it.

The Student Health Center—If you think you have a psychiatric or psychological problem—if you even *suspect* you might have a psychiatric or psychological problem—get an evaluation from the student health service or counseling center or a psychiatrist at home. Yes, you might be using depression or anxiety or insomnia or ADD as an excuse for not doing your work, but that doesn't mean you don't have the problem.

And you are not in a position to sort out, on your own, whether you have a psychiatric or psychological problem. You can't make a diagnosis from a Web site, by talking to friends with these problems, or by checking off symptoms on a checklist published in a magazine. More important, you can't *rule out* a diagnosis without a professional consultation.

You already know you can't make a medical diagnosis on your own. So why would you try to make a psychiatric diagnosis on your own? If you were unusually fatigued, would you try to figure out whether you had mono or anemia or hypoglycemia or MS or whatever by looking up the symptoms online or in a medical textbook? No, you'd go see the doctor. Would you tell yourself *I'm sure my symptoms are normal, they're no big deal, it's embarrassing to be sick,* or *it's humiliating to get help?* I would hope not. Would you feel that your fatigue was a sign of moral weakness or a character flaw? Would you feel stigmatized by going to the doctor or suspect her motives for taking your problem seriously and trying to get to the bottom of it? Would you resist her treatment suggestions because you thought she was too quick to start you on medication? Would you be afraid of becoming dependent on the doctor if she prescribed a course of treatment that required a number of follow-up visits? Of course you wouldn't.

Well, the same logic should apply to symptoms of depression, anxiety, inability to focus, insomnia, suicidal thinking, fearfulness, confusion, obsessing about your weight, hearing voices, and so forth. Go see the doctor.

All these psychiatric problems are treatable. But, left untreated, they make school very difficult. They interfere with your academic performance or your happiness or both.

Treating ADD makes studying and writing papers *dramatically* easier and more enjoyable. Treating depression, insomnia, OCD, anxiety, psychosis, and eating disorders: likewise.

I'll talk about these psychiatric conditions in more detail in later chapters. But, for now: go to the student health or counseling service at your college. And the student health center is a good place to start, because the professionals there have a particular interest, and a lot of experience, in treating college students. They've probably seen your problem or dealt with your issues a hundred times. They're less likely to dismiss or hype your complaint than a therapist in the community who sees students less often. Student health services generally employ an interdisciplinary approach, utilizing the special skills of a variety of different professionals, and they know all the resources available in the college community, which makes them better able to make an appropriate referral.

A Fork in the Road

If you've accompanied me to the end of this chapter, and tried to implement some of my suggestions (in which case you probably have the motivation and stamina to turn over a new leaf), but still can't get on track, you've reached a fork in the road. One path leads to more of the same—the slow, methodical, incremental attempt to improve your academic performance. The other path leads to a break from school.

Taking a break from school is not a decision you should make alone. You should talk it over with your parents, your dean, and, if you have one, your therapist. It's a tough path to follow because it means temporarily or permanently separating from your college friends, overcoming a (mistaken) sense of failure, and delaying graduation. But, if you're like the many, many students who've made the same choice, it may be the best decision you will make in your academic life.

Taking a break from school will give you the chance to reexamine your goals and your choices: Are you in the right college? Is college right for you, or is there another type of education that would better suit your aptitudes or prepare you for the career you want? Is there a psychiatric problem or learning disability that you've neglected for too long? Do you need more life experience or more time to grow up? Do you simply need a break after twelve or more years of school?

If and when you decide to return to school after taking a constructive break, you'll be more motivated, more skilled, more focused, and more successful.

Life is not a race, and it shouldn't be a painful ordeal. It's better to enjoy college and get something out of it than to graduate on time.

To quote Robert Frost from "The Road Not Taken":

> Two roads diverged in a wood, and I—
> I took the one less traveled by,
> And that has made all the difference.

Friendship

FRIENDSHIPS WITH INDIVIDUALS

If you're doing well academically, don't have other major problems, and have a few good friends, college will be pretty good. If you have a few people who like you and are on a similar wavelength, you'll be able to withstand homesickness, romantic disappointments, harsh winters, remote geography, a crummy dorm, maybe even a mismatch with your school. If you don't have friends, college will be tough.

The opportunities for meeting people in college are many and varied. They include orientation events, roommates, dorms, cafeterias, football games, sororities, fraternities, outing and other clubs, concerts, and collegewide events like homecoming. Most of all—since 60 percent of college students have jobs, including on-campus jobs arranged through the financial aid office—work is a great way to meet new people. If you then throw in lectures, study sections, and labs, it becomes nearly impossible *not* to meet people you could become friends with.

So how come you have no close friends?

Well, first of all, have you made the effort? You have to be honest with yourself about this because you'll probably be inclined to say yes even though, in truth, your effort has been perfunctory.

I've tried to make friends, you'll answer, but no one wants to make friends with *me*. And the people who are part of the group I hang out with seem to prefer each other's company to mine.

I'll address the challenge of getting into groups later. For now, let's focus on the challenge of trying to form friendships with individuals.

Forming a friendship is like committing a crime: It requires motive, means, and opportunity. Motive is why you want to have friendships in the first place. Means is how you go about trying to befriend the people you're interested in—what you do and what you offer. Opportunity is your receptivity to people and the initiatives you take to reach out to them.

Motive

There is only one durable motive for having friends—mutual enjoyment. No other motive—not mutual support or solidarity or loyalty or having a shared goal, shared complaint, or shared enemy—will produce friendship if the mutual enjoyment is missing. The actual focus of your shared enjoyment doesn't matter. Some of the best friendships grow out of a shared interest in an activity very few other people enjoy (experimental theater comes to mind). You want to have *fun* with the other person. This is true even if having fun involves something serious, such as politics, the environment, performing community service, running a co-op, or playing in a musical group. That friendship is based on mutual enjoyment is what distinguishes it from other kinds of relationships—teacher-student, business associate, or political ally—where there may or may not be affectionate bonds but where the primary motive for the relationship is a mutuality of interests.

If your reason for seeking friendship is something other than a desire for mutual enjoyment, and especially if your motive for friendship is therapeutic, you will approach relationships with the wrong attitude. You'll have a chip on your shoulder; you'll be angry with the other person for being insufficiently solicitous of your feelings; you'll be needy and demanding. If you have the wrong motives, you'll create a standard of friendship that is unrealistic and impossible for others to meet. You'll look for ways to prove to people that you're a "better friend" than they are (as if friendship were a competition): you'll buy them cards and gifts and go out of your way to listen to their problems because you want them to feel indebted to you, not because you care about them more than they care about you or, worse, to make them feel shabby when they don't reciprocate tit for tat. If your motive is mostly selfish rather than loving or sympathetic, you'll be wounded when the other person has failed to live up to your artificially high standards and use their failure to feel morally superior to them (when you actually feel *inferior* to them because you need *them* more than they need *you* or because you envy their insouciance). You'll take the opportunity to feel self-righteously indignant (because it gives you license to vent your anger over all of life's injustices). And you'll use the pretext of their "friendship failures" to preemptively end the relationship (before they discard you as too high maintenance).

Indeed, it is absolutely certain that your friends *will* fall short of your expectations in some way or another. Every friend will disappoint you sometime. But that doesn't necessarily mean she's not a good friend. If you're fond of her, and if you don't have unrealistic expectations, you'll be able to put her misdemeanors and shortcomings in perspective. You'll see the good in her and accept her on her own terms. You won't expect her to be exactly like you. You'll enjoy her in whatever way it's possible to enjoy her and not expect her to be all things to you. In short, you'll do for her what you'd expect her to do for you: you'll cut her some slack and give her the benefit of the doubt (or employ two other similar clichés having to do with making allowances).

The people I've seen who have the best friendships—who have many friends, who keep friends from every stage of their lives, and continually make new friends, who are liked by others and overcome conflicts with them—*like* people. They aren't oblivious to the idiosyncrasies and limitations of others (or of themselves), but they find a way to accept them as they are. They're no less competitive than others, but they don't let their competitiveness interfere with their appreciation of their friends. They're willing to deal with conflicts in the interests of strengthening the relationship, but they're not always spoiling for a fight. They're not paranoid; their default assumption is that most people *they* like will like *them* in return. If their friends are too busy to get together or call them less often than they call their friends, they don't feel rejected; they don't sulk or discard the friendship; they maintain it—but at an appropriate level of emotional investment.

People who have great friendships are able to do all these things, not because they're more confident or less sensitive than you are but because they enjoy other people more. They're not always hurt, offended, or angry. They're not thin-skinned. They don't expect perfection and they don't hold grudges.

Means

If your motive for friendship is mutual enjoyment, means and opportunity will be easy to arrange. You will find yourself more open to other people. Because you won't be feeling pathologically competitive with them, you'll be able to find them stimulating and enjoyable. You'll appreciate them, and they'll appreciate you in return.

The proper means for finding friends is to "be yourself" or just *a little bit better* than your normal self. Your goal, after all, is to be someone the other person finds enjoyable to be with, which can only occur if you're on the same wavelength. But the only way to determine whether or not you're on the same wavelength is by showing the other person who you are (except without all the negative stuff right up front—stuff that *might* be more appropriate to reveal later on).

Friendships have a natural history: They begin with the exciting discovery that you have a common bond—sense of humor, worldview, perceptions of other people, taste in music or movies, personal style, etc.—that isn't shared by everybody else. We all want to be spe-

cial, but, social animals that we are, it's still exciting to discover someone else who shares with us some of the traits that make us special.
That makes *them* special. And being special together makes it possible
for us to "get" them and vice versa.

Getting on the same wavelength can't be forced. It has to happen
more or less spontaneously. When you hit it off with someone, it
doesn't feel like work. Something about the other person allows you
to open up, to be more confident and less inhibited than usual. You
feel not just safer and more accepted but more interesting as well.
You feel appreciated for being your *true* self (which is just a little bit
better than your *usual* self).

Of course, that's the ideal. In reality, you don't always click with
potential friends right away. Sometimes it *does* take work. But how
much?

Well, it depends on whether *he* wants the friendship with *you* as
much as *you* want the friendship with *him*. And this is where something other than mutual enjoyment starts to play a part. This is where
concern about status (however defined), begins to rear its ugly head.
If you think he has a higher status than you, then your incentive to be
friends with him will likely be greater than his incentive to be friends
with you. You'll be more willing to "work" at the friendship than he
will—you'll be more tolerant of his faults and more forgiving of his
bad behavior than he of yours. (At least that's how it will feel to you.
You should try to keep in mind the possibility that he might not view
himself as having a higher status. Your perception of your relative
status may be entirely in your head.)

If your relationship with this person of real or imagined higher
status doesn't evolve in the direction of greater equality, however, you
may get tired of having to work harder at the friendship than he does.
You may still feel it's in your interests to maintain the connection,
but you'll begin to resent him. That's why the best friendships develop between people who view each other—or come to view each
other—as equals.

Knowing that equality is the basis of true mutuality won't cure you
of the desire to befriend people of higher status. The allure of such
people is almost universal. Of course, there are people who claim not

to be impressed by celebrity—and some of them may even be telling the truth. But for most of us there is something irresistible about people who, by virtue of their talent, intellect, beauty, style, wealth, or fame, stand out from the crowd. We want a connection with these standout people not only for the unseemly (though entirely understandable) reason that we hope their cachet will rub off on us but also because we imagine that they will be, as they often are, fascinating to be with—that they'll make our lives richer and more exciting.

So how do you go about making yourself attractive to someone you believe (rightly or wrongly) is above you in the social hierarchy? There are two ways: lowering the other guy's status or raising your own.

Lowering the other guy's status by pretending not to be impressed by him, or by pretending to be indifferent to having a friendship with him, is juvenile and phony. Still, it's surprising how often this middle-school ruse works—as long as the relationship eventually evolves in the direction of equality. If you have to keep pretending that you're doing her a favor by being friends with her, the effort involved in maintaining this facade will ruin mutual enjoyment—the true basis of friendship and cause the relationship to fall apart.

Raising your own status is a better way to go. But how do you do this? Most people will try to make themselves more interesting, more helpful, more sympathetic, and more entertaining than they might otherwise be. They'll work harder than they normally would to be appealing. They'll throw in goodies not offered by the competition—they'll do favors, they'll treat the other person to meals, they'll make themselves available at inconvenient times, they'll laugh harder at the other guy's jokes, and go along with activities that have little appeal. They'll try to be, not just *a little bit better*, but a *lot* better than their normal selves.

How should we feel about this strategy? Yes, it has the whiff of desperation, but is it truly demeaning? And can it lead to a real friendship down the road?

The answer to the question of how we feel about this strategy should be informed by empathy and understanding. After all, who of us hasn't been a little insecure when meeting new people or breaking into a new social circle? Who hasn't been a little too eager to find the other guy's lame jokes uproarious or his mundane opinions astonishingly insightful? Who hasn't tried to grease the wheels of friendship by going out of his way to help out a new acquaintance?

The reality is we've all gone out of our way to win over someone we admired and we've all benefited from doing this. So, no, working a little too hard to ingratiate yourself to a new friend need not be demeaning. And it *can* lead to real friendship. Of course, it would be better if the relationship evolved in the direction of equality. But more important is whether the relationship evolves in the direction of mutual enjoyment. If it does, then a true friendship will develop and the reward will be worth the effort.

Opportunity

Opportunity is what you do to increase the odds of meeting people you could be friends with. It involves both logistics—*where* to meet people—and receptivity—*how* to meet people.

The logistics are relatively straightforward: From the first day you arrive on campus (sometimes even before) you are thrown into contact with other students. There are the random mixing events provided by the school—orientation, roommate assignment, dorm assignment, meals in the cafeterias, classroom interaction, football games, and on-campus jobs—that rely on serendipity to produce a match. And there are the deliberate choices you make yourself—intramural teams, community service groups, clubs, extracurricular activities, sororities and fraternities, etc.—that rely on shared interests.

Both methods of meeting people are likely to produce at least a few hits, the college-initiated events because of their sheer profusion, the student initiated events because of their greater specificity. So, if you're not meeting simpatico people, the problem is not logistics, it's your lack of receptivity.

Receptivity is the vibe you give off that makes people feel comfortable meeting you. Having a chip on your shoulder, being chilly, aloof, or bored, is not a recipe for making friends. And that's true *even if you're acting that way defensively because you're shy.* New people are not required to make allowances for your bad behavior or to psychoanalyze you. It's your job to be friendly *despite* feeling anxious or insecure.

Social Phobia

Most people are a little anxious when they first meet new people. But their anxiety doesn't prevent them from making new friends. They fake being comfortable until they actually *feel* comfortable. People with social phobia can't do this. They're overwhelmed with anxiety when they have to meet new people, especially in a group. Unlike the ordinarily anxious, social phobics have such great difficulty attending parties or speaking up in class that they start to avoid these activities altogether.

Ordinary social anxiety is normal. Social phobia is not. If you're avoiding social gatherings, or courses where classroom participation is expected, because of paralyzing anxiety, you should seek psychiatric treatment. Social anxiety disorder is treatable with both psychotherapy and medication. College is too valuable to waste being afraid to socialize.

Obsessive Depression

Just as social phobia is different from (and much more intense than) mere shyness, obsessive depression is likewise different from (and much more intense than) mere self-consciousness. People with obsessive depression are not just self-conscious, they're so painfully self-conscious that they're actually self-absorbed. They're unable to relax enough to forget themselves and be in the moment. They're so convinced they're unattractive or undesirable that, even when they're with other people, they can't think of anything but themselves. Their mind is rarely free of analysis and regret: Did I say the wrong thing? Does he think I'm fat? Will she think I'm stupid? Am I having a bad hair day? Is he secretly mocking me?

If you're suffering from obsessive depression, no one can convince you that you're *not* unattractive or undesirable. You seize upon any real or (more often) imagined insult as confirmation of your pariah status, yet you dismiss every real compliment as faint praise or a white lie meant to appease you.

It's actually worse than that. Because part of you realizes that you're being neurotically self-absorbed, you hate yourself for your craziness as well. And that makes you hate everyone whom you imagine hates you for being that way! It's a mess: you're not only self-loathing, you loathe the world as well.

How do you break this vicious cycle of loathing and self-loathing? By eliminating the self-loathing. And the only way to eliminate the self-loathing is by treating the obsessive depression that underlies it. You can't do this simply by thinking positively or talking sense to yourself. If it were that easy, you'd probably already be cured. You need professional help. Overcoming obsessive depression takes either psychotherapy or, more often, a combination of psychotherapy and antidepressant medication.

When Friendships Fall Apart

You already know from your prior life experience that many if not most friendships end. They rupture because of a conflict that can't be resolved; they drift apart because of geographic separation, diverging interests, and the formation of new relationships that seem to have more juice. You outgrow friends, and they outgrow you. It's sad and it's painful—especially if you're the one who's been outgrown—but it's normal. Being on the receiving end of a breech in friendship feels like a slap in the face. If you're sure you've done nothing to warrant the change in status, you feel unjustly treated. It pisses you off. If you aren't sure whether you've done something to warrant the change in status—the usual case—it makes you angry *and* insecure.

Either way, the loss of a friendship feels like an injury, which makes you want to be made whole again, either by winning back your erstwhile friend or by spurning him in return. But sometimes the best strategy is to let go. Friendships end. It doesn't necessarily make you a bad person if you're the one who ends it; and it doesn't necessarily make you a victim if it's the other one who does.

"I'm Not Really a Very Nice Person"   Every now and then, I see a young person who is having a problem maintaining her friendships. She has little trouble making friends; her trouble is keeping them. After several weeks of gentle exploration, she will eventually tell me why: "I'm not really a very nice person. I'm competitive, touchy, envious, overly sensitive, petty and not very generous." Although she's not proud of the fact, she has to admit that she feels diminished by her friends' successes and secretly tickled by their failures. "I can fake it for awhile," she says. "But I live in dread of the fatal slip—the remark or action that reveals my true colors."

Of course, there is always at least a grain of truth to this kind of negative self-assessment. After all, who among us is incapable of being nasty, selfish and quick to take offense? And who hasn't coveted a friend's cool stuff or enjoyed a laugh at her expense? Because most of us are a mixture of selfishness and generosity, meanness and love, the answer is not many.

Fortunately, most of us manage to keep the dark side from overwhelming the light. On our good days the struggle isn't too difficult. But on our bad days, when we're feeling deprived and beleaguered, or lonely and desperate, it's harder to keep the balance from getting out of whack. Feeling unhappy tends to bring out the worst in us. And we know it. So even if we try not to let it show, we're sure others can see it in our behavior toward them, not least in our lack of enthusiasm for *their* happiness. A vicious cycle begins that we feel powerless to stop: our emotional stinginess makes us appear remote and defensive, which makes *others* begin to pull away. And *their* pulling away makes us feel hurt and resentful, which makes us even more awkward and withholding.

There are various places in the vicious cycle where you can intervene to stop it: you can make an effort to be more charitable and friendly to *the other person*—but if you were able to easily do that you wouldn't have been in this bad place to begin with—or you can try to stop the negativity by being more tolerant of *yourself*.

Being tolerant of yourself doesn't mean allowing yourself to be nasty or mean-spirited to others; it means accepting the bad thoughts with the good—while striving *in your behavior* to be good. It means being less harshly self-critical and more accepting of your own unworthy thoughts and feelings. This is important as a general principle, but it is particularly important when you're in a downward spiral of recrimination and bitterness.

Let's say you feel resentful of your friend because she's managed to get really thin and you're feeling fat. (I use this example because it's so common.) By being 1. less angry at yourself for being envious of your friend and 2. more forgiving of yourself for not being as thin, you will find that you feel better about yourself—hence less resentful toward your friend.

Most people who feel too negatively toward their friends also feel too negatively toward themselves. They tend to be just as harsh and intolerant of their own foibles as those of other people. Very often they have a long history of chronic, low-grade depression, which aggravates their perfectionism and causes them to be constantly unhappy with themselves. Once their depression is treated, their interpersonal problems will often disappear fairly easily.

So, yes, do try to *be* a good person. But if you're struggling to remain positive in your relationships with others, try to be more forgiving of yourself as well—and make sure you're not depressed. The best remedy for negativity is happiness.

"To Thine Own Self Be True"   Not everybody can be your best friend. You may be one of those quirky individuals who is truly close to only a few other people during your lifetime. There may be many people with whom you're able to have fun and with whom you have a few things in common, but, even with those people, you may never quite feel that you're on the same wavelength.

If you're different, but not *too* different, college can be difficult. You can *appear* to fit in without *really* fitting in. You're capable of *coming across* like a normal twenty year old who's comfortable with his peers. You're just not capable of actually *feeling* like a normal twenty year old—because you're *not* comfortable with most of your peers. You'll feel like a phony and wonder when you're going to get caught. You'll doubt whether anyone else feels the way you do and wonder whether there's something wrong with you that you can't genuinely enjoy your friends or believe they enjoy you.

In some ways it would be easier if you were too different from your friends to even go through the motions of fitting in. You'd know for sure you were out of the mainstream and be forced to accept it. You'd probably find it easier to make friends with the other "misfits" who *can't* fit in. But because you *can* fit in, you'll believe you're like everyone else—except less socially adept. Naturally, your self-doubt will grow, even as your ability to go through the motions becomes more seamless.

What to do? Well, the first thing to realize is that you're not alone. At least some of your friends will feel the way you do—they're on the periphery of the group and don't quite fit in either. So while it's true many seemingly mainstream young people are able to feel happy and in sync with their social environments, many are not.

The second thing to realize is that just because you haven't found a true bosom buddy—a friend with whom you feel a great affinity—it doesn't mean there's something wrong with you. If you're a person with unusual and special attributes, it stands to reason it will be more difficult for you to find someone else who can fully appreciate those attributes and whose attributes closely match your own. You may not find such a person in college. If you're lucky, you'll find that person in your spouse or life partner. Fortunately, as people mature and pursue occupations that reflect their individual preferences and aptitudes, it becomes statistically more likely that they'll come in contact with others who share their outlook and interests.

In the meantime, do your best to fit in. Develop your social skills. Accept that not everybody can be your best friend, but try your best to be friendly. There is a lot to be said for learning how to enjoy people who are *not* like you. But don't become discouraged if you have not yet found those few people with whom you can forge a deep lifelong friendship. If you can stay true to yourself, your faith will one day be rewarded.

FRIENDSHIPS WITH GROUPS

Birth of the Cool

If you're a college student, you're probably very familiar with the concept of shame. You're familiar with feeling red-faced, awkward, inadequate, embarrassingly flawed, and even a little weird—at least some of the time. You're also acutely aware of the importance of *concealing* your shame, of appearing, so to speak, *un*ashamed.

And what's the best way to appear *un*ashamed? By appearing to be cool. Cool, however, is merely the flip side of shame—not its true opposite. The true opposite of shame is being at peace with yourself, being more concerned with your own judgment than with the judgment of others. So being cool is not really the cure for shame, it's more the camouflage. And although most college students don't want to appear to be *trying* to be cool (cool, after all, being effortless), they at least don't want to appear to be *un*cool.

The desire to be cool—to be untroubled by insecurity, awkwardness, or unworldliness—begins when a person first becomes aware of sex. As Freud pointed out, awareness of sex, broadly defined, begins around age five—just when children are starting school and forming groups. But awareness of sex really takes off during middle school, when puberty and peer pressure first stir their toxic brew. Middle school (to reference the great jazz trumpeter, Miles Davis) is the birth of the cool. The death of the cool—at least nowadays—is death itself.

Fortunately, the desire to be cool—barring certain kinds of assaults on your dignity and confidence—becomes less powerful and less pervasive as you get older. Unfortunately, this admirable process doesn't start until *after* college. *During* college there are enough assaults on dignity and confidence to make George Clooney, Barack Obama, or even Michelle Obama feel uncool.

There are intentional assaults on your dignity and confidence, like orientation, frat parties, hazing, rush, and senior (or secret) societies. And there are unintentional assaults, like having to sleep in a noisy dorm and eat disgusting cafeteria food with a bunch of happy-seeming kids who've already made a million friends while you're still feeling at sea.

There are all the challenges of college that undermine confidence and well-being, like homesickness, loneliness, sleep disruption, and weight gain; there are academic pressures and disappointments; and there are the rejections, slights, and rebuffs that are inevitable in any social setting. And, of course, every school, from elementary to university, has a cool crowd whose sole purpose appears to be to stir up envy and hatred in everyone else.

In college there are a number of cool crowds. They form around outstanding academic achievement and high-value clubs and extracurriculars like the newspaper and drama club. They form around the frats and sororities and selective societies. And they form around the old reliables: beauty, money, and pedigree.

There are three ways to deal with the cool crowd: you can try to join it, you can feign disdain but secretly feel disgruntled not to be in it, or you can not give a damn and make your friends based on common interests and mutual affection. Needless to say, not giving a damn is the best approach, but it won't suffice if you believe you have the personal attributes to qualify for membership in the cool crowd. In that case, you'll feel torn: you'll want to join the cool crowd but be unsure how big a sacrifice of your dignity and emotional energy to make in order to apply for membership.

Not all cool crowds are equally obnoxious. In contradistinction to social cliques where unearned attributes—like class and connections—trump real achievements—like skill, effort, and commitment—inclusion in the elites that govern campus clubs, extracurricular organizations, and even fraternities and sororities is generally earned on the basis of seniority and merit. Leadership of the drama club, newspaper, or community service organizations is less likely to be awarded on the basis of a "beauty contest" than is leadership of a group whose principal agenda is organizing parties.

Of course, political acumen, charm, and personal appeal will always improve the fortunes of those who possess such traits compared to those who lack or eschew them. But this is as it should be. Finesse in dealing with people is not some manipulative ploy that substitutes for real merit and achievement. Finesse in dealing with people is an achievement in itself—and one that, unlike social class, can be cultivated by anyone who cares to make the effort. Nor is it merely self-serving: interpersonal skill fosters the greater good by making everyone feel valuable and included.

Learning how to be more socially adept doesn't mean that you have to become phony, hypocritical, or dishonest. (Doing that would make you not adept but manipulative—and rather transparently so.) It means making an effort to enlarge your sphere of sympathy to people *outside* yourself and your immediate circle. It forces you to increase your empathy and respect for the feelings of others and, in so doing, foster a climate of civility and belonging. Good manners, charm, diplomacy, friendliness, and politesse advance the interests of the group along with your own.

The microcosmic world of college offers an excellent opportunity to develop your interpersonal skills. And interpersonal skills are at least as valuable as any other skills in helping you to have a good life afterward. Finesse in dealing with other people makes you more comfortable with yourself and with the world. You shouldn't reject the opportunity to become more socially adept just because people in the cool crowd appear to be more talented in that sphere. Like most other worthwhile endeavors, social aptitude is 10 percent talent and 90 percent work.

Still, it is the way of the world that the naturally cool and comely will often have an unearned advantage over the rest of us in advancing their aims. And no group, no matter how humanistic, will be entirely free of this contaminant. In meritocratic groups, like the school newspaper, where you can work your way into the inner circle by excelling at the organizational mission—writing, reporting, editing, photographing, drawing, marketing, selling advertising, and publishing—the advantage of the cool and comely can be overcome by hard work. In social groups, like those that coalesce around a shared interest in popular culture, in-jokes, partying, and shopping, it will be harder to figure out how to become an insider. Don't assume, however, that the group should reach out to *you*. If you think you might like to be part of such a group, you have an obligation to reach out to *it*. You have to try to make the effort to participate in their activities, to resist becoming paranoid if individuals in the group seem initially more comfortable with each other than with you, and to avoid feeling rejected and then sulking if it takes time for you to gain full membership or if you never become a true insider.

It's important to keep in mind that college groups, whether formal or informal, are made up of college students—not Wall Street tycoons, movie stars, and aristocrats (at least not usually), but kids in their early twenties pretty much like you. Some have gone to exclusive private schools, have wealthy or famous parents, grew up in New York, Chicago, or Los Angeles, drive BMWs and Priuses, are plugged in to the hippest music, have the "correct" political views, and an incredible fashion sense. Some may even be talented in their own right. And that can be intimidating. But that doesn't mean they've managed to transcend human nature and are now free of the same kinds of insecurities and flaws that plague you. Nor does it mean they necessarily think they're better than you or that you couldn't possibly be friends with them.

Of course, it also doesn't mean that the cool kids are *obliged* to be friends with you. Friendships are voluntary, not contractual, and they don't exist to foster a progressive agenda. Although college provides a unique opportunity for social mixing, people with similar backgrounds and attributes tend to feel more comfortable with each other and stick together, as they do in the outside world. The cool kids are trying to create an accepting environment for themselves just like everyone else. Their groups are no more intrinsically exclusive than those that claim superiority based on musical taste or rigorous environmentalism. The only difference is that cool kids form clubs that people want to get into.

Gaining entrée to informal social groups that seem to have social cachet *may* make you feel good. But failing to gain entrée will *definitely* make you feel bad. Since the outcome of your bid for acceptance is sometimes uncertain and potentially humiliating, you may decide it's not worth the effort.

You may decide to improve your risk/reward ratio by forming associations on the basis of similar background and personal affinity, instead of on cachet.

Or you may decide to go further—you may decide to break out of the middle and high school model of social grouping and take advantage of the fact that you're in college. You get the chance to make a fresh start. Because you're forced to live and study alongside students of various races, ethnicities, religions, sexual orientations, socioeconomic and geographic backgrounds, college provides a unique opportunity to begin friendships with kids whose upbringings are different from your own.

Freshman year is probably the best time to take advantage of this opportunity. Everyone is new to the school, friendship groups have not yet congealed, and self-segregation in eating places, residences, frats, and sororities has not yet taken place. Of course, freshman year is also the time when you most want to create a home for yourself by finding people you're comfortable with—people who'll get your humor, style, and tastes: people who'll get *you*. And it's natural to assume you'll do this more easily with students from similar backgrounds with whom (you imagine) you have more in common. But, if you push yourself outside your comfort zone and try to get to know kids from different backgrounds, you might make a surprising and life-changing discovery. You might discover that you have more in common with a few people who are superficially *un*like you than you do with a lot of people who are superficially like you.

And that's really cool.

Portrait of the Artist as a Young Student

Not all groups are cool in the same way: some groups are cool in a conventional way; some are cool in an unconventional way. Both species of cool have their models in the outside world. The model for the conventional cool group is high society. The model for the unconventional cool group is the artists collective. Everyone knows that conventional social elites enforce strict norms. What may be less well known is that unconventional groups do the same thing—they have a set of rules, and those rules can be just as strictly enforced. If you have attitudes or behaviors that deviate from those norms—and most people do—you may feel pressured to suppress your deviant tendencies by presenting a fake persona to your peers and, worse, by suppressing a vital part of your own personality.

Jenny, a studio art major in her mid-twenties, was the victim of just such a process. She had become depressed during her sophomore year of college and been put on a series of antidepressant medications but had never fully recovered. By the time she came to see me, several years after graduation, she was so enervated by her depression that her voice was barely audible; it was an effort for her even to smile.

There were a number of factors, including a genetic predisposition, that had contributed to the onset of Jenny's depression. But an important one, which had been overlooked, was the influence of her fellow student artists.

Before falling under the spell of these young Virginia Woolfs and Jackson Pollocks, Jenny had been a vivacious, playful, self-aware young woman, confident of her attractiveness and social skills, who liked to wear makeup, dress stylishly, and go to clubs with friends. By the time she was finished sitting around with her fellow poets and painters discussing the sacrifices demanded by art, Jenny had become "serious," shy, and dowdy. She had lost her mojo.

It didn't help that her boyfriend of the time disparaged her stylishness and sex appeal, on the one hand, while cheating on her with "bimbos" (his word), on the other. (Though seemingly contradictory, it's not unusual for groups seeking liberation from "bourgeois society" to be both libertine and puritanical at the same time.)

So it made sense that Jenny continued to struggle with depression despite being on antidepressant medication: she was stifling the best part of herself—her elan, her passion, and her spontaneity. Worse than that, she had come to believe that those very traits—the wellspring of her confidence and creativity—were the greatest impediments to her artistic expression. She was convinced that she had to destroy what was unique and essential about herself in order to be considered a serious artist.

And she was losing the battle. A small healthy part of her spirit was rebelling against the tyranny of self-negation and struggling to find the light. She was failing to completely conquer the shallow, the frivolous, and the merely beautiful. So now she was depressed not just because she was *suppressing* her joy but also because she was *failing* to suppress her joy.

Yet it was precisely that failure—the struggle of her spirit to resist being conquered—that gave her the chance to overcome her depression. It took very little time in therapy for Jenny to realize that her friends' views on the need for artistic austerity had stifled her and undermined her confidence. She quickly understood that she had to "be herself" to be happy and creative, that the viewpoints of others were not necessarily superior to her own, and that she couldn't make herself conform to inimical views even if she wanted to.

In understanding herself better, Jenny began to understand the psychology of her friends better too. She realized, with empathy and compassion, that their motives were mixed. Yes, there was idealism and the search for truth, but there was also competitiveness and sexual politics. And sometimes competitiveness and sexual politics took on the guise of idealism and the search for truth. Her boyfriend hadn't made her insecure about her sophistication and femininity because they disgusted him as he had claimed; he had made her insecure about her sophistication and femininity because he was intoxicated and threatened by them and afraid she'd dump him if she realized how special she was.

It's hard to understand why Jenny didn't see all this at the time. Why didn't she just find a new group of friends and tell her boyfriend to go to hell? Why did it take Jenny three years of college and two years after college to break free of this damaging internal conflict?

One reason was shame. Jenny was ashamed that the very attributes that made her special were the ones most disparaged by the group. She came to believe that her style and vivacity were unacceptable in a "serious" artist—that they implied superficiality and a lack of deep creativity and had to be suppressed. Jenny's friends professed to believe that artists must renounce materialism and suffer for their art. And so Jenny suffered for her art.

The other reason it took Jenny so long to break free was love. Had she not been in love with one of its members, Jenny would probably have realized sooner that her personality was being stifled by the group. But, as it was, she couldn't break away from the group without breaking up with her boyfriend—and that was something she wasn't prepared to do.

Looking at Jenny's group from afar, we might be inclined to find their self-seriousness laughable. By trying to repudiate the sitcom sensibility of the wider culture, they were actually buying into one of its most enduring myths—that of the struggling artist at odds with society. But we shouldn't laugh. In a world where serious art is either marginalized or made into a luxury item for the very rich, developing an identity as an artist cannot be easy. These young people were not trying to be poseurs; they were trying to think like artists. And who knows? They might be right. It *might* be necessary for them to strip away the facile gratifications of middlebrow culture in order to find their voices amid the buzz of celebrity and the din of commercial entertainment.

So even if it turns out to be a passing phase, which Jenny's friends themselves outgrow and find amusing, we shouldn't mock their seeming pretensions. We should be as patient and supportive of the affectations of neophyte artists as we are of the affectations of beginning doctors with their white coats and dangling stethoscopes and of baby investment bankers with their Brooks Brothers suits and old-fashioned briefcases.

Unfortunately, Jenny's group of neophyte artists was unable to extend to her the same understanding that I'm advocating we extend to them. It wasn't their fault: they couldn't both repudiate and embrace the enticements and entitlements of materialism at the same time. No more could Jenny both challenge herself artistically and retain her old personality. It would have caused too much cognitive dissonance. But because Jenny was more vibrant and mainstream than the other members of the group, she had more to sacrifice—which made her internal struggle harder than theirs. And because her internal struggle was harder, she also experienced more shame about the difficulty of subordinating her innate exuberance to the group's harsh ideals.

Eventually, Jenny did succeed in suppressing her personality, but only at the cost of depression and emotional depletion. Whether or not Jenny's sacrifice will ultimately help or hurt her artistic expression, I can't say. I can say that, in the short run, it robbed her of her joie de vivre and sense of self. It turned her into a shell, and made her more tentative about her own creativity.

In trying to be "cool," Jenny lost her warmth. Many years were wasted before she was strong enough to reclaim it.

Minority Groups

Most students enter college expecting to enlarge their worldview, to have their beliefs and biases challenged, and to interact with classmates from different backgrounds. They may plan to affiliate principally with students from their own racial, ethnic, or religious group. But they usually hope to get to know students from other groups as well.

Most students enter college with an open mind but, regrettably, with their prejudices unexamined. Sometimes these prejudices are obviously negative: rich people are snooty, blacks and Hispanics are in this college only because of affirmative action, and Asians are good in math but poor in humanities. Sometimes these prejudices are negative despite *appearing* positive: people from the Midwest are nicer than people from the coasts (i.e., they're bland), blacks and Hispanics have more soul than whites (i.e., they're less intellectual), and Asians are more successful because they work harder (i.e., they're less creative).

The problem with prejudice, whether obviously negative or apparently positive, is that it forces people into a box—the box of group identity. Once in that box, people are seen not so much as individuals but as members of the group to which they've been assigned. And I do mean "assigned," because usually the most obvious trait is the one used to fix their group identity. Once in the box, their unique mixture of individual traits, even of heritages, is homogenized and replaced with one defining label: you're black, you're Latino, you're Native American, you're Asian, you're WASP, or you're Muslim. Never mind that you're also upper middle class, Dominican, have a French father, were born in Beverly Hills, are poor, or secular.

Of course, there are good reasons, both historic and contemporary, why individuals might *voluntarily* seek to identify themselves with a particular group. We don't yet live in a society free of racial, ethnic, religious, or gender prejudices. Membership in a group can help minorities overcome discrimination, provide solidarity and support, and celebrate differences sometimes devalued by the wider culture.

On a more mundane level, membership in a group also helps people of similar backgrounds feel comfortable and accepted—and this is true whether the group represents a minority or a majority of the population—although resentment may arise when outsiders are excluded or made to feel unwelcome.

There is also a big difference between *choosing* to identify with a group yourself and being *forced* to do so by other people. This applies (though to a lesser degree) even if the other people forcing you into the group are people *like* you, people *in* the group. Many students are content to affiliate mostly with classmates of the same racial, ethnic, or religious background—and they should be free to do so. But some students prefer to go their own way when it comes to choosing the groups they want to identify with—and they should be free to do so too.

Though by no means the norm, I have seen minority students criticized, sometimes cruelly, by their own racial, ethnic, or religious confreres for venturing too far outside the fold. I've seen a black student from Ghana harassed by some of her African American classmates for choosing to hang out with white students from her suburban high school instead of with black kids from the inner city. I've seen an upper-class African American man mocked by both black and white students for wearing preppy clothes and preferring classical music and jazz to hip-hop. I've seen modern Orthodox Jews criticized by their more liberal fellows for being too politically conservative and liberal Jews being rebuked by their Orthodox classmates for being self-hating. I've seen Indian men criticized by their Indian friends for dating Caucasian women and Chinese women criticized by their Chinese friends for dating African American men.

None of these efforts by "the community" to enforce racial, ethnic, or religious solidarity was malicious—indeed, most were motivated by a sincere desire to foster identification and fellowship and to provide mutual support. And although most students have the confidence to resist this pressure and befriend whomever they like, many students are troubled by it. They feel they've betrayed their roots or, worse, internalized the societal bias against their group.

The *desire* to affiliate with your own racial, ethnic, or religious group is normal, healthy, and educational. The *pressure* to identify with your own group—especially if it precludes making friends wherever you want—is harmful not only to your own development but to the very notion of diversity as part of a college education.

Take the Long View

It's important to take the long view of your social life. Friendships wax and wane over the entire four or five years of college. Groups form, reform, and fall apart. New groups form each semester. Clubs and fraternities evolve as freshmen arrive and seniors leave. Friends go abroad and return with new friends. Living arrangements change yearly, throwing together a whole new group of people. The cool crowd becomes uncool. And the people you wanted to associate with in your first semester will likely be different than the ones you end up being close to when you graduate.

Every college student goes through periods of loneliness and alienation, when past effort has come to naught and future effort appears futile. Every college student—every person—sometimes feels like a loser. Don't give in to despair. And don't give up. Many lifelong friendships are begun only in the final semester of college or even after graduation. Sooner or later, you'll make new friends, perhaps better friends, and find your niche.

Either way, within a year of graduation you'll have a whole new bunch of friends, and the travails of college will be largely forgotten.

Sex and Love

COLLEGE IS A HOTBED OF sexual activity: True or False?

Answer: False.

The American College Health Association–National College Health Assessment of 80,121 university students finds that 29.9 percent had *no* sexual partners during the prior year and 46.4 percent had only one. Hardly the orgy depicted in *Girls Gone Wild*. Though it should be noted that 10 percent of men and 6 percent of women claim to have had four or more sexual partners![1]

Still, that's not the perception. According to the same report, although 34.2 percent of students reported having had vaginal intercourse one or more times in the past 30 days, 94.6 percent *thought* the

---

1. American College Health Association, American College Health Association–National College Health Assessment (ACHA-NCHA) Reference Group Executive Summary, Spring 2008 (Baltimore: American College Health Association; 2008). These data can be accessed at http://www.acha-ncha.org/. Although this survey is updated annually, the numbers do not change significantly from year to year.

typical student had had vaginal intercourse in the past 30 days" (my emphasis).

In other words, college students think that *everyone* is having sex. And two-thirds think everyone—*but them*—is having sex.

So, if you're having sex—great. If you're not—don't feel badly about it.

What the statistics don't tell us is how enjoyable the sex is or whether it takes place within the context of a casual hookup or a loving relationship.

SEX

By the time students reach college, is there anything they don't already know about sex? Most college students have been having Sex Ed (if not sex) since middle school. They know—or can easily find out—nearly everything they need to know about genital anatomy, birth control, STDs, honeymoon cystitis, the HPV vaccine, HIV testing, and when to take the morning-after pill. They've been told that condoms are the best safeguards against STDs, but have discovered that they also diminish male sexual enjoyment. If they watch TV or go to the movies, they know that masturbation is normal but that Internet pornography can be addictive. They've been taught to think that homosexuality is a normal variant and that homophobia is bad—unless their religious training has taught them the opposite, in which case, if they happen to be gay, they don't know what to think. They've learned that casual sex is OK but that promiscuity—loosely defined (no pun intended)—is not. They've had it drummed into them that coercion of any kind is verboten and that drunkenness diminishes the capacity for consent.

Of course, *knowing* and *doing* are not the same things. Knowing about STDs doesn't guarantee that college students will always practice safe sex, and knowing about contraception doesn't mean they'll never get pregnant. But knowing does improve the odds of doing.

What college students *don't* know as much about is all the psychological stuff that goes along with sex. They know about oral, vaginal, and anal intercourse, but not necessarily whether they're comfortable performing them. They know about erections, lubrication, and orgasms, but not whether they always occur or what it means if they don't. They know that foreplay and consideration for their partners' satisfaction is desirable but not where to draw the line between giving and getting. They know that sex and love can be separated, but not if, or when, they should be.

They don't necessarily know how to reconcile their religious and moral beliefs with their desires or whether their hang-ups are reasonable and a reflection of healthy self-esteem or silly and the result of unanalyzed neurosis. College students don't know whether the kinky acts that turn them on or that they see on pornography sites are "sick" or merely adventuresome.

These internal conflicts are true for every student, but they are particularly true if you're trying to come to grips with being lesbian, gay, bisexual, transgender, or queer. College may be the first chance you've had to explore your sexual identity and orientation without the weight of your parents' expectations or the pressure of your childhood community. But with newfound freedoms come new choices: Should you come out to your family and friends or pursue your relationships in private like straight people get to do? Should you affiliate mostly with other-gendered students and become involved with LGBTQ politics and culture or live openly according to your own lights without self-identifying?

It's a lot to ask of an eighteen or twenty-two year old—especially where the relevant information is so confusing—to reconcile feelings so intense and conflicted and come up with answers to questions so complex. But there is no choice: No one else knows better than you how *you* need to reconcile these feelings and answer these questions. And no one else has to live with the consequences.

Your parents and friends and therapists may know how *they* feel about these questions—more likely they know how they *ought* to feel about these questions—but what they can't know is how *you* should feel about them. Even I can't help you with these questions. You will have to sort them out for yourself.

What I *can* tell you about these questions is that you should trust your own feelings. In fact, I think you have no choice but to trust your own feelings (even though they're a moving target that will continue to shift over a lifetime) because to do otherwise is to declare war on yourself. And the worst thing you can do, and the most painful, is to be at war with yourself—to try to be something you're not, or to feel something you don't, just because it's the "normal" or expected thing to be or feel. You have to be who you are—and be at peace with that. This is not a destination most people arrive at in college; but college is a good place from which to begin the journey.

You may believe, for example, that you ought to be sexually open-minded and willing to experiment. You may wish to please your partner or avoid his disapproval. You may wish to be sophisticated and a good lover. You may want more than anything in the world to be "normal." But what you should not want to do is go against your strongly held taboos, push yourself too far outside your comfort zone, or feel ashamed of your inhibitions or inexperience. You will figure out what you like and don't like, and those preferences may continue to evolve as you gain maturity and experience.

Certainly, you have an ethical duty to avoid behaviors that are risky or harmful. Not every desire or impulse has to be—or should be—expressed. Not every request made by your partner has to be fulfilled. Taking advantage of your partner's emotional vulnerability or intoxication to pressure her for sex or forcing yourself on her is immoral and perhaps criminal. Hurting yourself or your partner (I mean for real), or allowing yourself to be hurt (for real), is wrong. This is true whether or not sex is involved, but, because sex is so intimate and emotionally freighted, *when* sex is involved, hurting or being hurt is especially harmful.

Other than that, it's a bit tricky to determine what constitutes normal sexuality. People don't talk honestly with each other about their sexual practices. They especially don't talk with each other about the sexual practices that embarrass them. But, based on many decades of survey data and many centuries of erotic art, the range of sexual practices is both pretty wide and pretty narrow.

Problems of Arousal

One thing that will always be true is that your partner's arousal (even if it's only in a masturbatory fantasy) will be arousing to you. Which means that the best way to turn on your partner is to show him or her that *you're* turned on.

But what if that *doesn't* happen? What if you can't become aroused? As a man, what if you can't get or maintain an erection? As a woman, what if you can't get lubricated enough or relaxed enough to permit painless intercourse?

Well, first of all, let's try to avoid making the problem worse by hyping it. Nearly everyone—regardless of age—is let down by his genitals sooner or later. The reason for this is that your genitals are connected to your brain. Most of the time the minds of college students are controlled by their genitals but, every now and then, their genitals are controlled by their minds. When this happens, even college students may be unable to "get it up." They may *want* to have sex but, because they're nervous, because some silly little thing is intruding on their arousal, or because they're trying too hard to impress or to please, they may not able to get aroused enough to do so.

One not so little thing that has become a bone (pardon the pun) of contention in the AIDS era is the use of condoms. Between arranging to have them available (which implies the expectation of intercourse), fumbling to get them on, and the decrease in stimulation they produce, condoms—though absolutely necessary until you are in a committed relationship with a partner whose STD and HIV status you know—are a downer.

This problem of "mind over matter" will only become a "dysfunction" if 1. you think of it as a dysfunction and start worrying about it every time you attempt to have sex, 2. you think of sex as a test of masculinity, femininity, or technical prowess, 3. if you subscribe to the theory that the only legitimate goal of sex is intercourse, or 4. you purge your mind of arousing thoughts during sex because you believe your thoughts are "dirty" or otherwise unacceptable. (This is a good time to remember the distinction between thoughts, which can go anywhere, and actions, which can't.)

If you accept that "stuff happens" to everyone—that even healthy, horny young people can fail to become fully aroused—and if you don't try too hard to overcompensate, you may be able to avoid "performance anxiety" in the future. And if you realize that the goal of sex is intimacy and pleasure—not prowess in performing one particular act—you may be able to enjoy sex without always feeling pressured to have intercourse.

Of course, as a backup for men there are Viagra, Cialis, and Levitra and for women there are lubricating gels, dilators, and vibrators. Soon, perhaps, there will be drugs to enhance female sexual response. Once that happens, "frigidity" (lack of arousal) and vaginismus (painful vaginal spasms that block penetration) will lose their stigmas too.

Because Viagra and its sister drugs make getting an erection almost foolproof, many men *without* erectile problems use them for casual dating "just in case." It should be noted, however, that Viagra can produce *too* big an erection—yes, there is such a thing—which may, paradoxically, diminish sexual pleasure. When taking these drugs for the first time, it's a good idea to start with a low dose.

While I don't think college students should use Viagra drugs in anticipation of a problem, I do think they should use them early enough to nip an erectile problem in the bud. Just knowing that they *could* use Viagra may be all that's needed to prevent performance anxiety from taking root.

Although sexual difficulties are more obvious in men, they are actually slightly more common in women (43 percent versus 31 percent by some estimates). That this should be the case is understandable—vaginal intercourse is a bigger deal for women than it is for men. Here's why: 1. the lining of the vagina is more delicate than the skin of the penis, which means that women are more susceptible to injury and STDs during intercourse than men; 2. penetrating is intrinsically more "aggressive" than being penetrated, which means that being the "bottom" in intercourse requires a higher degree of trust than being the "top"; 3. condoms can break and diaphragms can get dislodged, which means that pregnancy is a constant fear for women who aren't taking the pill, even when they're using other methods of birth control. Fortunately, the morning-after pill is now widely available over the counter—although it has to be used with seventy-two hours of unprotected intercourse.

Women who are having persistent problems getting aroused, who are unable to relax enough to permit vaginal intercourse, or who have pain when they do should see their gynecologists. These problems are common, and most gynecologists will be familiar with their causes and treatments.

Premature Ejaculation

Premature ejaculation—ejaculating before intercourse is initiated or sustained—is a common problem, especially in younger men. Like all sexual dysfunctions, it's not just frustrating, it's embarrassing because it leads the man to worry that he isn't satisfying his partner. Indeed, "not being able to satisfy my partner" is the great nightmare of men (and, to a lesser extent, women) with problems of arousal or the ability to sustain intercourse.

Premature ejaculation tends to occur less frequently the more time you spend with the same partner. This is of little help, however, if you're starting a new relationship or just trying to hook up with people casually. Not having confidence in your ability to function sexually, whether due to problems of arousal or orgasm, can lead to avoidance and shame.

So how to deal with premature ejaculation? Some men masturbate before a date to reduce their sexual tension and some try to distract themselves during sex to reduce their arousal. Sex therapists, however, recommend the opposite: on the theory that you have more control over a reflex when you pay attention to the incoming sensory data, they recommend *focusing* on the sensations in your penis during arousal rather than trying to ignore them.

If none of these techniques work, do not despair. There is help in the medicine cabinet. The SSRIs, like Paxil, Zoloft, Lexapro, etc., produce delayed orgasm as a common side effect. Paxil, for example, taken a few hours before sex in doses as low as 10mg, can help reduce premature ejaculation. You and your doctor can experiment with the choice of medicine, dose, and timing, based on your response to the drug and side effects. No doubt there will soon be medicines available specifically for premature ejaculation, just as there are for erectile dysfunction.

One problem that can result from too strenuous an effort to prolong intercourse is delayed or inhibited orgasm. Delayed orgasm has a number of causes, but trying to "last" in order to satisfy your partner is one that can be easily remedied. You should not try to satisfy or impress your sexual partner if doing so will result in loss of erection, vaginal irritation, inhibited orgasm, or boredom.

Sexual Wisdom

Part of the responsibility of being a considerate lover is learning about your partner and teaching your partner about you. And, since everyone is different, it's not always obvious what those preferences might be. It isn't fair to expect your partner to be able to read your mind. Most men, for example, still hope to achieve mutual orgasm with their partner during vaginal intercourse even though many, if not most, women are anatomically unable to do so without direct clitoral stimulation. That's not chauvinism; it's ignorance. Which is why the key to good sex is not masterly technique but patient and respectful communication.

The goal of sex is pleasure and, sometimes, intimacy. It is not a test of desirability, virility, or sexual prowess. I know it's hard not to feel a little pressured at the beginning to prove that you're not a rank amateur and that you know how to satisfy your partner. It's hard not to compete with imaginary rivals who've either been to bed or will go to bed with the person you're currently making love to. And it's hard not to feel ashamed if you feel you've frustrated the woman or man you're trying to favorably impress. But keep a few things in mind: 1. Almost everyone has sexual problems at one time or another. 2. Having a sexual problem doesn't mean you're undersexed, confused about your sexual orientation, not attracted to your partner, or lacking in sex appeal. It probably just means you're trying too hard. 3. Most sexual dysfunctions improve with time or when you're in a safe relationship with a trustworthy partner. 4. All sexual dysfunctions can be treated—so don't be embarrassed to seek treatment from your doctor.

And finally, if your partner is having a sexual problem, be understanding. Don't take it personally. Don't overreact. His difficulty is not a reflection on you—or even on him for that matter. It doesn't mean he finds you unattractive. It doesn't mean she doesn't like you. It doesn't mean he's being selfish or hostile. It doesn't mean she's frigid or hates sex. All it means is that we are human. Sex is not an unconscious animal reflex but a complex human interaction that involves thoughts and feelings.

The best way to deal with sexual difficulties, whether in yourself or your partner, is with low-key patience and levity.

LOVE

If there's one gender stereotype that has persisted more or less intact through fifty years of feminist scholarship, and plenty of evidence to the contrary, it is that females are more romantic than males—that females want relationships and males want sex. Even among gay men and women—arguably the most progressive and gender-bending communities in our culture—the myth of a masculine/feminine difference when it comes to romance continues to be honored in the breech.

So who am I to demur? Yet, in my experience, males are just as likely to want relationships as females, and females just as likely to want sex. And, if there is a difference between the sexes, it's statistical rather than individual. Were it not so, most romantic couples would consist only of women, and most sex would be had only by men. Perhaps *on average* men wait longer to fall in love and have relationships than women. But, sooner or later, both women and men—at least *most*—want to settle down and find a mate.

And when men and women fall in love, find a mate, or move on, the course of their relationships, like all good stories, has a beginning, a middle, and an end. The beginning and end are more emotionally fraught than the middle. But all the parts, from beginning to end, are tortured and wonderful, each in its own way.

The Beginning

"Play the field." "Take it slow." "Don't get all hot and heavy right away." "Date a lot of people before you settle down."

That's the romantic advice most young people get from their parents before going off to college. And it's great advice: it increases the probability of making a good choice of girlfriend or boyfriend, and decreases the probability of getting a broken heart. Too bad nobody can follow it.

At least nobody *in their early twenties* can follow it—which is probably why well-meaning adults feel compelled to give it in the first place. Yes, one day, when you've had your heart broken a few times by lovers unwisely chosen, you *might* be able to "take it slow." But, at your age, when falling in love is so new and the demands of reality so distant, once you really like someone, it's virtually impossible *not* to be head over heels.

So I'm not going to advise you to take it slow or play the field—it would be unrealistic and possibly shaming to do so. I'm going to try instead to examine a few of the issues that arise once you've already fallen for someone.

Attraction

In the ideal world, we'd all be attracted to people who were perfectly suited to us. (In which case our parents' advice about playing the field would be unnecessary.) We'd value people who were stable, loving, and kind more than people who were mercurial, sexy, and cool. We'd be more attracted to the sweeties than the hotties, the good guys than the bad boys. And we'd choose those who like us as much as we like them instead of those who like us more or less.

Of course, we don't live in the ideal world—we live in the real world. And, in the real world, narcissism casts a stronger spell than caring. Elusiveness is more intoxicating than availability. Novelty is more fascinating than familiarity. And looks are more alluring than character.

For all sorts of reasons—some crazy, some sensible—in the real world the "wrong" choice is often more attractive than the "right" choice. And although the young are more susceptible to this perverse logic than the old, the old are not immune either.

So how is it that half the married population eventually ends up making the right choice? Generally, it's because they get attracted to someone cute, sexy, and cool who turns out *not* to be narcissistic, fickle, or cold. Or, better still, someone adorable, loving, and good gets attracted to them—and they're in the right frame of mind to respond positively when it happens.

Being in the right frame of mind, however, takes confidence, experience, and maturity—traits most college students don't yet have. What you, as a college student, *do* have, though, is idealism and hope. You may not be prepared to make the compromises that adults are prepared to make in order to find a life partner—but you don't need to, because you're not yet at that stage. You're allowed to make choices that are more dreamy and passion driven than adults because, whatever your marital fantasies, you're not likely to end up being stuck with those choices. You don't have to find a girlfriend or boyfriend who has *all* the important traits; you can find one who has a few in spades. Getting involved with the "wrong" person is not only a prerogative of college life, it's the means by which you gain the requisite confidence, experience, and maturity to make the right choice later on. (It's also the means by which you learn to cope with rejection and loss.)

So here's the bottom line in assessing the traits of a boyfriend or girlfriend:

Consistent, loving, generous, honest, reasonable, intelligent, happy, forgiving, flexible, self-aware, responsible, makes you feel good about yourself, beautiful inside as well as out—*good*.

Moody, angry, cold, selfish, slippery, unreasonable, ignorant, tortured, unforgiving, rigid, not self-reflective, irresponsible, dishonest, makes you feel insecure, beautiful outside but ugly inside—*bad*.

Make the best choice you can. But when you fail—and you will—don't be too hard on yourself. Everyone is a fool for love. And everyone makes mistakes. Just don't make the mistake permanent by marrying it.

The Middle

Being in a loving, stable, committed relationship is wonderful. You know what you're going to be doing Saturday night; you can have sex whenever you want; you have the dignity and status of being someone's boyfriend or girlfriend; you're less likely to get an STD.

Knowing that someone loves you makes it easier to love yourself. I know that *you have to love yourself before you can love anyone else.* But the truth is it's harder to love yourself when you feel lonely and can't get a date than when you have a lover who thinks you're smart and beautiful. Being in a good relationship is more therapeutic than five years on the couch with Freud. Conversely, being in a bad relationship can make you feel like a total loser.

What is a good relationship? A good relationship is one where you can be yourself and feel good about it because your partner "gets" you—accepts and loves you for who you are. Conversely, a bad relationship is one where you can't risk being yourself for fear of being ridiculed, attacked, or rejected.

To paraphrase Tolstoy, happy relationships are all alike: they're easy. (Unfortunately, for our Tolstoy reference and for life, all *un*happy relationships are alike too: they're hard.) Now I know that you have to be prepared to "work" at a relationship, that relationships don't always run smoothly, etc., etc. But in good relationships the work is easy: the problems are small, differences can be easily ironed out, nobody stays angry for long, both people are prepared to compromise, communication is open and direct, nobody tries to "win" arguments at the expense of seeking to understand the other person's point of view. Most important, there is trust. There is no game playing; there is no fear that the other person will cheat; there is no need for jealousy. There is no drama.

How do good relationships happen? They happen because both partners are good people who are sane and have the important things in common.

Bad relationships result from the reverse of all the conditions that make good relationships good. Bad relationships are hard work, and the work never gets easier. There is a lack of goodwill and trust—usually for valid reasons—which leads to a high quotient of insecurity and unhappiness. That the unhappiness is interrupted by moments of ecstatic bliss—reconciliations after explosions or infidelities, unexpected kindness after cruelty, and makeup sex—is what keeps bad relationships going.

Maybe because the lows are lower in bad relationships, the highs seem higher. Or maybe because the highs are a form of intermittent reinforcement, "making the relationship work" becomes compelling. Whatever the reason, getting out of a bad relationship is actually harder than getting out of a good one.

College Commitments

Let me introduce a note of realism to my discussion of good and bad relationships and ask a question. Is it realistic—not desirable but *realistic*—to expect young adults in their early twenties to have the same level of integrity in their dealings with their romantic partners as we expect from adults? Is it realistic, for instance, to expect college students to refrain from hooking up with a cute girl or boy when their girlfriends or boyfriends are away for the summer or studying abroad? Could it even be *desirable* for them to do so? And if it turns out *not* to be realistic to expect complete fidelity during absences, is it at least realistic to expect college students to be honest with their partners about these dalliances once they're back together?

The answer, I believe, is no to the former but yes to the latter. No, because I think it's unrealistic to expect college students to be completely faithful to their boyfriends or girlfriends during extended breaks. (I'll explain why in a moment.) But yes, because I think it's realistic to expect college students to at least be honest with their partners about those dalliances.

Let me begin by making an obvious point: the love relationships of college students are less critical and less likely to be permanent than the relationships of adults who are married or contemplating marriage. I'm not condoning infidelity in college students. I know that you can be just as intensely in love, feel just as ready to get married, and be just as easily hurt as older adults. And I know that respect and empathy are traits that ought to be present from childhood on. But, realistically, are the stakes as high for college students as they are for married couples or couples contemplating marriage? Do we even *want* the stakes to be as high? Don't we want young adults to be able to have experiences that will help them mature? Don't we want them to be able to move in and out of relationships more easily than later on?

I think the answer is yes—provided they do so with consideration for the other person and, above all, with honesty. And that's where personal character and integrity enter into the picture. It may not be realistic, or even desirable, to expect college students to cleave to each other as if they were a married couple. It *is* realistic, I think, to expect college students to deal honestly with each other. If you're going to be separated from your boyfriend or girlfriend for an extended period of time, I think you should discuss, in advance, what level of fidelity you expect from each other. You should endeavor, if possible, to forewarn your partner of your desire to see other people. You should be prepared to come clean about any dalliances you have. And you should be honest with each other about the fact that infidelity, even if agreed to in advance, may bring about the demise of the relationship and, at the very least, cause great pain and leave permanent scars.

What do you do if it's clear that the person you've had four or five dates with is more into the relationship than you are. She hasn't explicitly asked you whether or not the relationship is monogamous—because doing so would be premature—but it's clear that she's starting to view it that way. Are you allowed to play dumb and avoid dealing with the question until she brings it up directly? Are you obligated to apprise her of your feelings all along the way?

This is a tricky one. Not all communication is verbal. The person you're dating may not want to ask you explicitly where you stand for fear of pressuring you or scaring you off. That doesn't mean she doesn't want to know. Should you volunteer the information and risk hurting her feelings unnecessarily, making her angry or losing her? Can you simply say you haven't made up your mind yet?

And what obligation does the *other* person have? Isn't she an adult just like you? Wouldn't it be patronizing to take responsibility for her feelings instead of relying on her to protect her own interests? If she really wants to know how you feel, isn't it up to her to ask? And, if she hasn't asked, does that free you from a requirement to make your feelings clear?

What to say to the person you're dating, and when to say it, is a judgment call. But it should be guided by several principles. You should always be considerate and tactful, but you should never lie. You're not required to disclose every vicissitude of your feelings, but you shouldn't try to communicate your ambivalence by being cold or mean. You're not obligated to make a commitment you're not ready to make, just because the other person wants you to, but you're not allowed to lead him on when you know you're not smitten just because you like the companionship or sex. You don't have to be a saint, but you do have to be a kind and decent person.

Above all, whether you're the one more into the relationship or not, you have an obligation to be honest.

Being honest isn't easy. It isn't easy to be honest with the *other person* when doing so might entail causing him pain or losing him altogether. It isn't easy to be honest with *yourself* when doing so may entail facing up to the fact that you're more attached to her than she is to you. It's hard to inflict pain on someone you care for, and it's hard to walk away from a relationship, even if you know the relationship will continue to cause you frustration and pain. But being honest is the only thing that allows you and the other person to exercise free will—to continue the relationship with trust or to end it with dignity.

The End

Breaking up is good to do. It's the only way to get out of an unsuitable or unsatisfactory relationship and to avoid marrying the wrong person.

Breaking up, as we all know, is also hard to do. And it's especially hard to do when you're breaking up with someone you love.

Given the biological imperatives of self-preservation and reproduction, it shouldn't be surprising that we're hardwired to form strong attachments. Still, it's humbling to realize that, no matter how sophisticated and rational we think we may be, the act of falling in love, and the act of breaking up, are so strongly governed by biology. If breaking up is hard to do, falling in love is sometimes too easy to do. And both can make you feel as if you've been overcome by an illness.

At times breaking up *is* an illness: You can't eat; you can't sleep; you can't think about anything but her. Every song or place reminds you of him; every corny ad on television makes you cry. You want to call or e-mail her but you know you shouldn't; you want to find out what he's doing and with whom he's doing it. You feel lonely and jealous and empty and unlovable. The future seems devoid of possibility and the present scarcely worth living. Were it not for the fact that the cause is obvious, you'd think you were clinically depressed. And sometimes, if you can't get over your grief at the loss of the relationship, if you can't stop obsessing about your lost love, if you're unable to function at school or enjoy your friends, you *may* be depressed. (In which case you should seek professional help.)

It's true of breakups as of other awful experiences that "what does not destroy me makes me stronger." You will never be quite as torn up by future breakups as you were by the breakup of your first true love. Having survived a painful first breakup, you will feel braver in the future about ending relationships that aren't right for you. Having survived a painful breakup is empowering. But knowing that the pain is making you stronger won't make you feel better while you're going through it. That's why so many people, despite their better judgment, keep going back to their old boyfriends and girlfriends. They say yes, yes, yes when their friends tell them they're being stupid to continue the relationship, but no, no, no when it's time to say the final goodbye.

Bad relationships are kept going by fear—fear of loss and fear of being replaced: *I know I'll never find anyone as wonderful as Brad to love me. But Brad's so cute, he'll be with somebody else by tomorrow.* And bad relationships are also kept going by hope—hope that things will get better: *I know Kimberly flirts with other guys. But if she really knew how much it hurt me, I'm sure she wouldn't do it.*

So what is it that finally drives a stake through the heart of a relationship? What puts the dying beast out of its misery? Well, after all the false endings and endless rationalizations, the heartfelt apologies and tearful reconciliations, the thing that usually brings a love affair to its end is not wisdom and strength but exhaustion. You're sick of the emotional ups and downs; you're fed up with the other person's nonsense; most of all, you're utterly and completely bored by your own angst. You are so *over* it.

Either that or you meet someone else.

Depression and Suicide

DEPRESSION: THE CHICKEN OR THE EGG?

Although doing poorly academically is the biggest reason college students come to see me, it's not the problem they usually present with. The problem they usually present with is depression.

Jody, a twenty-one year old who came to see me during her Christmas break, is typical. Because of a dropped semester, she was half way between her junior and senior years.

"I've been in treatment for anxiety and depression for five years," she announced. "But the symptons never seems to go away."

"My bad mood is causing me trouble at school because all I want to do is sleep. I sleep all day long and then I'm up all night—so I miss a lot of classes."

Despite her irregular attendance, Jody was managing to scrape by in school, but without much enthusiasm and with mediocre results. She had been in psychotherapy for depression for years and had tried virtually every antidepressant, with only temporary benefit. Inevitably, after each new medication, the depression and malaise returned. Jody's mother had sought me out as a last resort (rarely a promising beginning).

In my experience, most depressed college students who are doing poorly in school are depressed because they're doing poorly, not the other way around. But in Jody's case there was an interesting wrinkle: her depression had begun in high school after a rejection by a boy.

"I fell into a deep depression," she explained. "I stayed up all night, crying and obsessing about the boy. I felt humiliated and refused to go to school or even to go out."

(Part of the difficulty in trying to sort out whether or not a person is "clinically" depressed—especially someone like Jody who has been in therapy for a long time—is that they use the word "depressed" to mean everything from "very unhappy" to "near-suicidal.")

After the breakup with her boyfriend, Jody missed several weeks of school completely. After her return, she missed one or two days a week. Her academic performance, which had been excellent before the rejection, became lackluster.

Jody's parents had taken her to a psychiatrist who had, quite correctly, diagnosed clinical depression and started her on Lexapro. Her depression improved, but not completely, and she continued to oversleep, miss a lot of school, and fight with her worried parents.

Despite the decline in her grades, however, Jody got into a good college and planned to turn over a new leaf once she started there. But, daunted by the college workload and feeling homesick, she reverted to her old habits and began to skip classes. Her grades suffered, so, naturally, she felt anxious and depressed. A psychiatrist at school changed her Lexapro to Effexor and started her on Adderall for presumptive ADD, Lamictal for mood-swings, and Klonopin for insomnia and anxiety—again with equivocal results. By the time she came to see me she was on four medicines and still not feeling normal.

I asked Jody what her ambition had been before her problems started. I could tell she was unhappy with herself, and I sensed that the biggest cause of her depression might be the possible loss of her childhood dream and hopes for a bright future.

She told me that since childhood she had planned to become a pediatrician, treating children with cancer, like her mother who was an oncology nurse.

"With the grades I have now, I'll never get into medical school," she opined. "I have no idea why I'm even *going* to school at this point. I just want to get through."

"Maybe I'll go into fashion design," she continued. "I have a good eye for what people look good in."

I asked Jody whether staying in bed, skipping classes, and feeling depressed was a way of trying to deal with her disappointment in herself. She agreed.

"You learned in high school that depression was an acceptable reason for avoiding schoolwork," I explained. "And you've continued to use that tactic—to be 'depressed'—in college."

Jody took up my point. "I think my depression may just be a bad habit," she admitted. "Which is why the antidepressant medication isn't really working. The real problem is I've stopped trying and I'm not happy with the results."

I encouraged Jody to come up with a goal that would give her a renewed sense of purpose and to do her best to attend classes.

We also agreed that, despite the lack of evidence that it was helping, Jody should remain on her medication until the end of the term.

"When you come back in the summer," I told her. "We'll try to taper you off the medicines. More important, we'll see if you can give up the habit of using 'depression' as an escape from responsibility."

"You're a bright young woman. There's no reason why you can't get back on track and have a great life."

After the Christmas break, Jody returned to school and managed to pass her spring semester. But in early June, immediately after the end of school, Jody took a trip to Israel, with a group of young people from her church, that changed her life.

Because of the early mornings and long days, the inspiration of visiting ancient religious sites and sharing a deeply moving experience with like-minded students, Jody began to reestablish a healthy image of herself.

After the trip, with my encouragement and supervision, she tapered off her antidepressant medication. By the time she returned to college in the fall, Jody was a new person—her old predepressive self. She had a renewed sense of discipline and purpose. She changed her major to religious studies, attended all her classes, enjoyed the intellectual stimulation of her courses, worked hard, and ended her college career with a flourish.

One difficulty in trying to help students who are floundering academically is that the factors that produce or aggravate laziness—like ADD, substance abuse, mood disorders, etc.—can also be produced or aggravated *by* laziness. Sometimes you can't sort out whether the problem is causing the poor academic performance or the poor academic performance is causing the problem. In most cases, each is causing the other.

This is a particularly vexing conundrum because of shame. Oddly enough, many students feel less ashamed of being given a diagnosis of depression, substance abuse, or ADD than of being labeled lazy. A psychiatric or learning disability diagnosis, because it's beyond your control, seems to absolve you of responsibility for your underperformance, whereas laziness, because it's volitional, does not. And because therapists can treat psychiatric and learning disorders but not laziness, they (we) are only too happy to make the diagnoses and start the psychotherapy and, sometimes, the meds.

The plot thickens when the student has a bona fide psychiatric disorder, especially depression, which *does* interfere with academic work. Then the problem can become a vicious circle: the depression interferes with performance and the poor performance aggravates the depression—which, in turn, aggravates the poor work effort and so forth. Since depression is comparatively easy to treat these days, evidence that the work avoidance is leading to the depression instead of the other way around becomes apparent only when the depression refuses to go away with proper treatment.

Jody's example is typical of these treatment-resistant cases of putative depression. She's a bright and able student who presents to her psychiatrist with all the symptoms of a major depressive disorder following a painful loss. She's (appropriately) given antidepressants and psychotherapy but, two months or two years later, still has symptoms of depression and still can't manage to do her schoolwork. Her depression symptoms are more resistant, stickier, more nebulous and pervasive that ever, and she is much more debilitated by them than one would expect. She and her parents are becoming increasingly desperate and irritated with each other. And, though they're afraid to say so, they all now suspect that her depression might have become an excuse for avoiding school and, more broadly, adult life.

In circumstances like these it takes a brave therapist to refrain from giving yet more treatment for depression and to begin dealing with the underlying fear, avoidance, and shame. The student is afraid you'll label her a malingerer and give her parents ammunition with which to chastise her. The parents are afraid you'll blame them for their child's problem—for putting too much pressure on her or for some other inadvertent child-rearing misdemeanor. The psychiatrist is afraid of missing a true biological mood disorder. And what all three are afraid of is that a promising young person will end up a lifelong invalid.

Psychiatrists are not the only therapists capable of making the honest mistake of mislabeling work avoidance as psychological illness. Nonpsychiatrists are just as likely as psychopharmacologists to want to delve into the "root causes" of the depression rather than encourage the student to return to school and to confront his fears and avoidance techniques as they arise there. It pains me to say this, but, sometimes, if the choice is between therapy that perpetuates the myth the student is disabled, because of untreatable depression, or no therapy at all—no therapy may be better. With no therapy, the student can at least avoid creating an excuse for himself about why he's unable to return to school or, later, get a job.

Best, of course, would be a two-pronged approach: appropriate medication that eradicates the student's treatable impediments to fulfilling his potential and good psychotherapy that supports his attempt to return to school and that tactfully and nonjudgmentally confronts his avoidance of work.

It's worth looking for a therapist who has the maturity, confidence, and insight to recognize and treat the *actual* problem, rather than a therapist who "does what she does," regardless. You're more likely to find such a therapist, however, if you've already had the courage to recognize that your depression may be secondary to your floundering, rather than the other way around.

Psychiatric Medication

Quite a few young people arrive at college already on medication. There are several reasons for this. Many valid psychiatric conditions, including some very common ones like depression, panic attacks, drug abuse, and eating disorders, have their onset in the late teens and early twenties. Psychiatry has become more adept at managing even serious conditions on an outpatient basis. And, last (and this is a good thing), psychiatric problems are continuing to lose their stigma. Partly, this is due to the fact that the latest scientific research has established a "medical" basis for these disorders, which makes them no different from illnesses like diabetes or arthritis. And partly this is due to the fact that young people today are being more candid with their friends about being bipolar or depressed or anxious, and each succeeding generation seems to be generally more open and tolerant.

Having said that, our old friend shame still rears its ugly head. Too many college students are still hesitant about acknowledging and seeking help for emotional and psychiatric problems. This shame is *itself* a shame. All these conditions are treatable and most of them, when properly treated, are compatible with attending college and having a successful life. Untreated, however, they can be quite debilitating—making school and postschool life, at best, an uphill grind and, at worst, nearly impossible.

I will cover a few of the common psychiatric disorders confronted by college students just to give you some idea about, and alert you to, the possibility that you may be dealing with one of them. I do not intend to give you the means to make the diagnosis or to spell out all the modalities available for treating them. The DSM diagnostic criteria for these disorders are readily available on the Internet, from the American Psychiatric Association and other sources, or in the library. The danger of trying to diagnose yourself from the Internet or from something you read, however, is that you will use the criteria to convince yourself you *don't* have a problem or that you will be unduly affected by the disinformation or anecdotal experiences of a few vocal, usually disgruntled, patients who love to express themselves online.

If you think you might be depressed, anxious, paranoid, perplexed, or having trouble sleeping, eating, focusing, etc., you should seek a consultation with an expert trained to diagnose and treat these problems. Don't just talk to a friend or your abnormal psych professor about your problem. Go to the student health center or call your doctor at home and get a referral.

I don't want to say too much about treatments either. There are plenty of places to look up information about drugs and therapies that are better able to stay current, and go into greater depth, than I can in this book. And treatment, like diagnosis, should be prescribed by somebody with objectivity and clinical sophistication—i.e., not you.

I do, however, want to say something about psychiatric medication in general because there continues to be a resistance to prescribing and taking drugs for mental disorders not only among the lay public but even among some physicians.

Why is this so?

Let's begin by agreeing that psychiatric medication, like all medicines, should not be given without a clear indication and that only physicians who are knowledgeable about their risks and benefits, and can properly monitor them, should prescribe them. Let's also agree that most people would prefer to use more "natural" treatments if such treatments were shown to be safe and effective.

Both these caveats, of course, apply to *all* medications, not just those used to treat psychiatric conditions. The resistance to psychiatric medications, therefore, must entail something more.

One source of resistance to psychiatric medication in particular is the notion that mental conditions are different from bodily physical conditions. They are thought to be due to negative childhood experiences, psychological trauma, or a bad current situation—not, in other words, to some aberration in the chemistry or anatomy of the brain. Sometimes, even often, this is true. But there is a large body of reputable scientific evidence—from epidemiology, genetics, brain imaging, animal research, and clinical trials—showing unequivocally that many of the important disorders psychiatrists treat *are* due, at least in part, to an aberration in brain structure or function. There is also considerable evidence that even disorders that began as the result of some unfortunate life event—trauma, loss, disappointment, grief, or illness—can become autonomous of their original source and devolve into brain disorders that respond to medication. This seems entirely logical when you consider that everyday learning and memory involve permanent changes in brain chemistry.

Some people resist taking drugs by turning the idea that psychiatric conditions are like other medical conditions on its head: *If I don't take medication,* they reason, *then my condition isn't medical. And, if isn't medical, then it can't be very serious.* There's a name for this kind of reasoning: it's called denial.

Another source of resistance to psychiatric drugs in particular (as opposed to medications in general) is the worry that they may eventually be shown to cause brain damage. Some people who took first-generation antipsychotic drugs, like Thorazine and Haldol, for many years *did* develop a neurological condition called tardive dyskinesia. So the fear of permanent effects on the brain is not unreasonable. But all the commonly prescribed antidepressants (including the SSRIs like Lexapro and the tricyclics like Tofranil) and antianxiety medicines (including the benzodiazepines like Klonopin and Xanax) have been around long enough for signs of brain damage, or other permanent side effects, to have become apparent. And none have been reported.

Although second-generation antipsychotic drugs, like Zyprexa, Risperdal, and Seroquel, can have serious metabolic side effects, none, so far, have produced permanent negative effects on the brain. There is even animal model and epidemiological evidence emerging that suggests some psychiatric drugs, like lithium, may have a *protective* effect on the brain. Nevertheless, the newer and more novel the drug, the more cautious you should be about taking it for long periods.

Another concern frequently voiced by patients is the fear of addiction. This is because some psychiatric drugs, like the stimulants Ritalin and Adderall and the Valium drugs and sleeping pills, can cause dependence and sometimes be abused.

Dependence, however, is not the same as addiction. Drug dependence entails withdrawal (return of symptoms when the dose is lowered too quickly) and tolerance (loss of efficacy when the dose is increased too slowly). Addiction entails dependence *plus* abuse—drug-seeking despite adverse consequences and overuse or misuse of the drug for purposes other than those for which it was intended.

Antidepressants, mood stabilizers, and antipsychotic drugs do not produce dependence, let alone addiction. And even the stimulants, antianxiety drugs, and sleep medications, where some loss of efficacy is common over time, rarely cause addiction when properly prescribed and monitored. Unfortunately, Adderall, Klonopin, and other drugs you share with your friends are *not* being properly prescribed and monitored. And, although they are relatively benign most of the time, they can cause adverse reactions, interact badly with other drugs or alcohol, and even be abused.

Finally, there is the concern that psychiatric drugs will cover up the "real" problem, like a Band-Aid, making it harder to cure by psychotherapy or some other means. This concern is related to the erroneous notion that psychiatric disorders are not really medical illnesses, which I've already discussed, and to the laudable desire for self-reliance, which I commend. Most clinicians agree, however, that treating psychiatric illnesses with medication *reduces* some of the hurdles to successful exploration of psychological problems and makes it easier to undertake life changes. Treating psychiatric illness with appropriate—repeat: appropriate—medication makes the person *more* self-reliant, not less.

Depression

The problem with depression is that, to the depressed person, it often seems to make sense. *Of course I'm depressed,* she says to herself, *I'm behind in my work, I received a D on my midterm, my dog died, my parents are having problems, my boyfriend dumped me, my roommate stays up till all hours and keeps me awake, I binged on junk food, and now I'm premenstrual. You'd be depressed too if you had my problems.*

Well maybe, maybe not. It *is* true that someone facing those problems might feel miserable—for a while. It is *not* true that she would necessarily become depressed. The difference between everyday misery and real depression is that depression persists beyond a couple of weeks and begins to seep into a variety of social, mental, and physical functions. Depressed people experience an uncharacteristic erosion of happiness, confidence, optimism, resilience, motivation, and mental and physical energy. Their desire and ability to enjoy their friends, hobbies, work, recreational activities, and even sex starts to wane. If it gets bad enough, they may lose their appetite (or start to pig out), have trouble sleeping (or getting out of bed); they may even be plagued by fantasies of dying or killing themselves.

In terms of intensity and speed of onset, depression can feel like a nagging toothache, like a snapped femur, or like the expected death of a loved one. And it doesn't always appear in a pure form. Very often it's mixed with anxiety. The most painful form of depression is accompanied by "agitation"—a state of compulsive and entirely futile worrying that destroys your mental peace and makes the thought of killing yourself seem frighteningly appealing. In agitated depression, your thoughts become negative, and you replay things you "wrongly" did or said over and over again like a broken record. While you're obsessing, you may find yourself pacing around the room, wringing your hands, scratching your scalp, picking at your skin or your cuticles, jiggling your leg like a hyperactive schoolboy, or wanting to cut or burn yourself just to feel something different. And because the compulsive worrying is worse when you're not distracted by other activities—when you're trying to go to bed at night or when you wake up suddenly at 4:00 A.M. with your mind already churning—you walk around all day feeling exhausted yet unable to relax.

The capper to all this obsessing and negativity is that it makes the depression seem sensible—you *deserve* to feel depressed: you've offended your best friend, disappointed a professor, antagonized your parents, or stopped exercising and eating sensibly. Which is why depressed people in general, and college students in particular, don't get professional help for their depressions soon enough. They don't think they're capital D Depressed, they think they're understandably and appropriately small d depressed.

But, here is the important point: *even* if your depression seems to make sense—if you believe your depression was provoked by a real-life calamity or even by your own laziness, selfishness, stupidity, or bad judgment—it doesn't mean that it shouldn't be treated. Because whether or not your depression *seems* to have a cause is immaterial. What matters is whether it persists and whether it's adversely affecting your life. Clinical depressions tend to become autonomous of their putative causes and self-perpetuating. In other words, once triggered, depression can take on a life of its own, dragging you down long after the event that caused it has faded in importance.

Not all depressions are severe, of course, but even mild depressions can change the trajectory of your life. This is especially true for college students who are at an early stage of their lives and have not yet developed their careers or formed long-term relationships.

Imagine, for example, that your childhood dream was to become a doctor, but, because of depression, you couldn't concentrate well enough to ace organic chemistry. If you weren't depressed, you might decide to repeat the course during the summer and try to get a better grade. But, if you *were* depressed, you might decide—perhaps wrongly—that you were simply unable to handle the academic demands of medicine, and abandon your dream altogether.

There are plenty of other ways to be happy and fulfilled besides becoming a doctor, of course, but giving up on a long-held dream, especially when it may not have been necessary to do so, can lead to many years of sadness and regret.

Since many career paths begin in college (including some, like business or journalism, that may take place outside the classroom), psychiatric conditions occurring at this critical stage of life can not only undermine your ability to succeed but, worse, destroy your courage even to try. The road not taken in college, because of depression or other remediable problems, can end up pushing you permanently off track.

What to do? First, get help. If you are feeling down, becoming discouraged, and losing confidence—or are thinking of giving up on your dream—go to the student health service and talk to someone. Ask them whether they think you might be depressed. You should do this even if you think the reason you're depressed is that you're not doing well academically. You might be doing poorly academically because of depression, or the depression may have broken free of the original cause and become self-perpetuating.

If they tell you at the student health service you're depressed, allow them to treat you or refer you for treatment. Treatment consists of antidepressant medicine, psychotherapy, or both. Do not be afraid of either modality of treatment. Modern antidepressant medication is generally well tolerated, doesn't change your personality or interfere with performance at school or work, is not habit-forming, and begins working quickly—often within a week (though it might take several weeks to really take hold). Psychotherapy can be effective for moderate depressions by itself and is perfectly compatible with psychopharmacology. But if you are not starting to feel substantially better within a couple of weeks of starting psychotherapy, or if your improvement stalls, you should consider the addition of medication. At the very least, you should not reject the medication option out of hand or view it only as a treatment of last resort.

If you go to see a therapist and she tells you she *doesn't* think you're depressed, *but you think you are*, trust your own assessment and seek a second opinion. There still are too many therapists who think that if a depression "makes sense" it should be treated lightly or not at all. If you could afford the luxury of months of dithering before being properly treated, your symptoms were relatively mild and you already had a career, you might be able to hobble along without it screwing up your life. But, if you're a college student, you have neither the luxury of time nor the security of an established life to coast on. If you're a college student, you should insist on getting properly treated from the very beginning.

Once you're feeling back to normal—which can take a month, sometimes longer—you'll be in a better position to determine whether the real life issues you were grappling with were the cause or the consequence of your depression—and better able to make rational decisions about your future. This is the time to come to grips with your academic problems rather than hiding behind the depression to avoid dealing with them.

Because most antidepressant medication is safe and well tolerated, many nonpsychiatric physicians believe they are competent to treat garden-variety depression—and in simple cases they are. But the clinical challenge in treating all but the simplest cases of depression is not making the diagnosis and prescribing the medication but knowing when the patient has *fully* recovered and whether the dose is adequate to achieve full recovery.

Many nonpsychiatrists, in my experience, stop treating the patient before he's completely back to normal. The patient says, "I feel better," and the doctor says, "Great. Keep doing what you're doing." This is unfortunate, because many people who say they're better may only be *relatively* better, not *all* better.

Patients who are not thoroughly treated—who are not *all* better— have a higher rate of relapse and chronicity than those whose symptoms are totally eradicated. And because they think they're "better," partially treated patients continue to be adversely affected by residual symptoms without realizing that depression is still the source of their problems. They go back to erroneously attributing their residual depression solely to life events again. So, unless you are 100 percent back to normal (or, if you've been depressed most of your life, *better* than normal), you should see a psychiatrist with expertise in mood disorders.

And you should stay on the full therapeutic dose of your medicine until you're instructed to taper off. After you've been feeling well for a while, it will be tempting to reduce your dose of medicine or taper it off on your own. It will seem like a straightforward decision, particularly if you've already "forgotten" to take it for several days without any ill effects or your prescription has run out. You may want to save the expense of a final visit or avoid being talked into staying on medicine. But the decision about whether and how to go off a drug you've been prescribed for a psychiatric condition is not straightforward. You should consult with the doctor who put you on the medicine before going off it.

Suicide

Every year an alarming number of college students attempt, or die by, suicide. Because serious medical illnesses are fortunately rare, suicide is one of the leading causes of death in people your age. Most suicidal students are suffering from depression, but all, in some way or other, feel hopeless about continuing with their lives: they may feel ashamed about disappointing their parents, angry with their girlfriends or boyfriends, or experiencing such mental turmoil that they can't imagine getting relief in any other way. Some may want to punish the people they believe should have loved them better. But many are in the grip of a quiet despair in which they imagine their loved ones will be better off without them.

Since suicidal thoughts can cross the mind of nearly anyone during moments of frustration or unhappiness, when should you take these thoughts seriously? When should you talk to someone—a parent, a doctor, or, if no one else, a professor or friend—about them?

The correct answer is *every* time. It is not always easy, even for a psychiatrist, to discriminate between suicidal ideation that is worrisome and suicidal ideation that isn't. It's nearly impossible for someone in the grip of suicidal ideation (like you, if you're feeling suicidal) to make that distinction.

Certainly, you should consult a professional if your suicidal thoughts are frequent, recurrent, or persistent. They may be a symptom of depression. You should seek help immediately if you're spending time contemplating the method of killing yourself, have access to highly lethal means such as guns or a large store of drugs, and especially if you have a plan. If you're thinking of jumping or composing a suicide note, go to the emergency room, stat!

You should seek help if suicide feels like a welcome relief or if you're feeling agitated. You should seek help if you feel indifferent, cold, or numb about dying. You should seek help if you're picturing your family or friends reading your suicide note, finding your body, or attending your funeral. You should seek help if you're using drugs or alcohol frequently or if you're on prescription medications like Accutane for acne, interferon for hepatitis C, or steroids, hormones, amphetamines, or antidepressants that can sometimes increase the risk of feeling suicidal. You should seek help if a family member has attempted or completed suicide or suffered from a serious mental illness. You should seek help if you've attempted suicide before yourself.

If you've taken an overdose or injured yourself, call 911 and open the door to your room. Most people who survive a suicide attempt are relieved that they didn't succeed. Whatever misdemeanor you feel you've committed—a personal failure, a shameful act, or an interpersonal blunder that hurt someone or resulted in a humiliation to yourself—it is not a capital crime. Death is not a fitting punishment. You will feel very differently about your predicament very soon. Live and make your life, and the world, better.

Get help. Now.

Anxiety and Insomnia

ANXIETY

There is no bright line between anxiety and depression. Depression is often accompanied by anxiety, and anxiety can evolve into depression.

Anxiety, like depression, can be a signal that something is wrong. Anxiety that is short-lived, manageable, and appropriate is the mind's way of alerting you to an imminent danger. Anxiety that is persistent, hard to cope with, unwarranted by the degree of peril, and unrelieved by improved circumstances may be evidence of an anxiety disorder. In anxiety disorders, the symptoms of anxiety are either too great in absolute terms or out of proportion to the imminent danger in relative terms.

How do you figure out whether the anxiety is warranted or overblown? How do you know whether you're appropriately anxious or having the symptoms of an anxiety disorder? Consider the three *I*s: intensity, intractability, and interference. If the anxiety symptoms are *intense* (intolerably severe), *intractable* (don't dramatically diminish or disappear with passage of time or change of circumstances), and *interfere* with your ability to function optimally, then you have more than normal anxiety.

I'm not including as a criterion whether or not the anxiety has an apparent cause. That's because, where anxiety is concerned, there's *always* a cause, especially if you're a college student—it's the end of semester crunch, your boyfriend won't commit, your parents are divorcing, or you're pledging an exclusive sorority. Even when there really isn't a cause (a true impending danger or overwhelming stress), it's human nature to find one: you're worried about a terrorist attack, you think your cold might be H1N1 flu, or you're preoccupied with climate change. If identifying a "cause" meant anxiety were normal, then there would be no such thing as abnormal anxiety. *All* (well, almost all) anxiety, including the anxiety of anxiety disorders, appears to have a "cause." So the issue is not whether the anxiety has a cause but how much distress and disability the anxiety is causing.

For example, nearly everyone feels *some* anxiety when he has to give a presentation in class or walks into a party where he doesn't know many people. If you have social anxiety disorder, however, you will be nearly *paralyzed* by the prospect. You'll look for excuses to avoid giving your talk altogether or drink heavily before going to a party.

The exception to the "no real cause" rule is post-traumatic stress disorder (PTSD) where there is *always* a real cause of the anxiety symptoms. In PTSD the cause is a significant trauma—combat, rape, severe accident or injury, direct exposure to a crime or terrorist attack, etc.—that threatens life and limb or overwhelms the mind's capacity to cope.

Panic Attacks

Panic attacks are the paradigm case of abnormal anxiety. They differ from ordinary anxiety episodes both quantitatively and qualitatively. Imagine how you'd feel if a man with a gun burst into your room. You'd feel as though you were about to die. Your heart would race and pound in your chest. You'd feel sweaty, dizzy, and nauseated. Your thoughts would race and become confused. And you'd be terrified that you might scream, faint, choke, lose control of your bodily functions, have a heart attack, or go crazy. That's how people with panic attacks feel when they're sitting on a subway car that has stopped between stations, when they've stayed up too late and consumed too much coffee studying for an exam, or, more commonly, when there is no apparent reason at all.

Not all panic attacks have all the symptoms I've described. But they are certainly unlike anything you will have felt before. They may only last for a few minutes, but they leave you shaky for hours afterward. If panic attacks recur, as they do in panic disorder, you begin to worry about when the next one will hit. And your baseline level of anxiety increases until, eventually, you feel anxious all the time.

Abnormal anxiety comes in a variety of forms. Besides panic disorder, there are generalized anxiety disorder, obsessive-compulsive disorder, social anxiety disorder, PTSD, and a number of less common diagnoses. If the anxiety symptoms are severe or persistent, they can lead to phobias—the avoidance of places or situations that aren't really dangerous but feel dangerous in the context of the irrational fear. Panic attacks lead you to avoid places—such as subways, elevators, bridges, restaurants, theaters, and crowds—where you'd feel trapped. Social anxiety leads you to avoid situations—such as speaking in front of your classmates in a large seminar, attending the first meeting of a club or fraternity, or auditioning for an improv group— where you'd feel exposed and potentially embarrassed or humiliated (by blushing, stammering, or having your mind go blank).

Fortunately, most anxiety disorders are highly treatable. As with all other illnesses and problems, however, the earlier you intervene, the easier it is to turn things around. If your anxiety is interfering with your academic work, your relationships, or just your sense of well-being, go to the student health service. Don't be mollified by reassurances that your anxiety is normal or appropriate given the stress you're under. Don't be put off just because your anxiety seems to have a cause. Anxiety that doesn't dissipate with reassurance or a reasonable change of circumstances should be treated with psychotherapy, medication, or both.

Psychotherapy

Psychotherapy for anxiety disorders comes in two forms: behavior modification (including cognitive behavior therapy—CBT) and exploratory psychotherapy.

Behavior therapies focus directly on symptom reduction. They provide tools for lessening the symptoms of anxiety (meditation and relaxation techniques) and for challenging the cognitive distortions that make everyday risks and dangers seem extrathreatening. When phobias have developed, behavior therapies gradually expose you to the situations you've been avoiding so that you no longer feel restricted by your anxiety. Most behavior therapies are time limited, say twelve to fifteen visits; many follow a treatment manual and involve homework assignments.

Some people find behavior therapies a bit boring or simplistic, but, in experienced hands, CBT, for example, can be quite dynamic and motivating. The nice thing about behavior therapies is that they deal directly with symptoms, and you can learn to apply them on your own and after you've completed therapy.

Exploratory psychotherapy, sometimes called psychoanalytically-oriented or psychodynamic psychotherapy, attempts to examine the meanings and psychological origins of anxiety. By uncovering the sometimes surprising reasons for your anxiety, exploratory psychotherapy helps to solve the riddle of why your anxiety is out of proportion to the circumstances that are apparently triggering it. Once you know *why* you're feeling anxious, your rational mind will help you to put your current stressors into perspective and reduce your symptoms.

Exploratory psychotherapy is more like what you see on television shows or in the movies. It's more interesting and complex than the behavior therapies, which makes it appealing to people who want to understand themselves as much as they want to get relief from their symptoms. Done well, exploratory psychotherapy can be efficient and productive. Done poorly, it can be frustratingly slow at producing either insight or symptom relief.

If you're psychologically minded, want to understand yourself, have subtle, long-standing symptoms that don't need immediate relief, exploratory psychotherapy may be for you. If you're not particularly interested in knowing *why* you're anxious, want to have concrete tools for suppressing your symptoms, and need pretty immediate relief, behavior therapies, like CBT may be a good place to start.

Providing you've given the initial treatment a chance to work (and had the chance to openly discuss your concerns about it with your therapist beforehand), you can always switch to a different modality of treatment (or therapist) if you feel you're not getting anywhere.

Medication

Modern psychiatry believes in treating the whole person, which means tackling the biological as well as the psychological and social causes of problems. While psychotherapy targets the psychological and social causes of anxiety, medication is uniquely effective at dealing with the biological component. And if you've ever experienced a panic attack, you'll appreciate how helpful treating the biological component can be.

As with psychotherapy, medication to treat anxiety comes in two forms. There are the benzodiazepines, like Klonopin, that quickly suppress the symptoms of anxiety, but also quickly wear off. And there are the antidepressants, like Zoloft and Lexapro, that take a week or more to kick in, but then tend to keep the anxiety symptoms at bay.

Both classes of drugs have their pros and cons. The benzodiazepines, like Klonopin, Ativan, Xanax, and Valium, give rapid temporary relief from mild to moderate anxiety but not usually from panic attacks. They are sedating, especially early on in the course of treatment, but don't produce sexual side effects or weight gain. Because drugs like Klonopin and Ativan tend to lose a little efficacy over time, resulting in the need for one or two dose increases, many clinicians and patients worry, often unnecessarily, about addiction. Used carefully under supervision for bona fide anxiety disorders, benzodiazepines are safe and effective. And unlike other drugs used for anxiety disorders, they can be used on an as-needed basis when the symptoms arise rather than every day.

Drugs like Zoloft and Lexapro, which began their lives as antidepressants, are uniquely helpful in blocking panic attacks and in controlling symptoms of obsessive-compulsive disorder (OCD). They're also helpful for social anxiety disorder and generalized anxiety disorder. Many clinicians are more trepidatious (perhaps excessively so) about using benzodiazepines than they are about using SSRIs because of the risk of dependence. But the SSRIs and other antidepressants have their own set of issues in treating anxiety: 1. They don't give immediate relief from symptoms the way benzodiazepines do, which means they sometimes have to be combined with a benzodiazepine at the beginning anyway. 2. They may actually cause a temporary flare-up of anxiety symptoms when they're first introduced, which means they have to be increased to a therapeutic level slowly. 3. They have to be taken daily, even after the symptoms have abated. 4. They can cause weight gain and sexual side effects (diminished libido and difficulty achieving orgasm) in some patients.

Fortunately, both classes of medication are very effective, which makes their cost/benefit ratios very favorable for treating anxiety disorders. Both types of medication can be combined with both types of psychotherapy. And, because of the symptom-relief they provide, both types of medication make the two types of psychotherapies go more smoothly.

Heidi had her first panic attack during spring break of her senior year. She didn't know it was a panic attack at the time. She just knew something was terribly wrong.

"I woke up feeling kind of blue," she explained. "Then, when I was having breakfast, I felt a sensation in the back of my neck that ran down my right side. My stomach felt like it was in a vice, and I started to cry."

"The symptoms went away after about twenty minutes," she continued. "But I got scared that I was really, really sick. I have irritable bowel syndrome, but the stomach pain was worse than anything I'd ever experienced with my IBS. My mind was racing. I was sweating a lot and I couldn't eat."

"I didn't have another episode until after I returned to school," she added. "Two weeks into the term, while I was reading over my senior thesis in preparation for discussing it with my adviser, the symptoms returned, but this time much stronger. I thought I was having a heart attack. Luckily, my roommate was home, and she took me to the hospital. The doctor there took a history and did a physical and an EKG. When she was finished, she told me I was having a panic attack."

"What treatment did the doctor recommend?" I asked her.

"She gave me Xanax," Heidi explained. "It has actually helped a fair amount, but I'm taking 0.25mg three times a day and it's making me too drowsy to work. I can still feel the symptoms coming on—I get racy and sweaty and start to panic—but they go away before it gets really bad."

"Have you had any more depression?" I asked.

"After the attacks occur I feel depressed for days," she answered.

Heidi told me that her mother always complained of palpitations and had gone to the emergency room on several occasions believing she was having a heart attack. Nevertheless, her mother had not been treated for panic disorder or for heart disease.

Heidi's baseline level of anxiety had gone up as a result of her panic attacks, but she had not developed any phobias. I confirmed the diagnosis of panic disorder and recommended the addition of Lexapro.

"We'll start the Lexapro at a low dose and increase it slowly," I explained. "Sometimes, if you increase the dose too quickly, it can cause a temporary flare-up of your anxiety symptoms. So, until the Lexapro is at a therapeutic level and begins to take effect, we'll keep you on the Xanax. Eventually, you'll be able to taper off the Xanax and be on Lexapro alone, which will be less sedating."

I explained that Lexapro can sometimes lower your sex drive and make it harder to achieve orgasm and that it can cause modest weight gain as well.

"Right now you might not care about the side effects because you just want relief from your panic attacks," I told her. "But in a few weeks, when you're feeling better, you may be more upset by the side effects and be tempted to stop the medication. If so, please don't be afraid to discuss your thoughts about the medicine with me. Going off the medicine prematurely increases the risk of relapse. And going off it abruptly can produce withdrawal symptoms."

"How long will I have to be on the Lexapro?" Heidi asked.

"For *at least* six months after the panic attacks have gone away," I explained. "And unless you're having bothersome side effects, you may want to stay on it for a year or longer."

We set up a series of weekly appointments. But before our first follow-up meeting, Heidi phoned me three times to clarify some small errors in the history she'd given me and to review some minor details of her diagnosis and treatment. People with panic disorder require a lot of reassurance.

Heidi also had a theory about why her first panic attack had occurred when it did. She explained that reading over her thesis had triggered an association to a professor she'd had in her sophomore year who had told her that she shouldn't major in sociology, the very field in which she was doing her thesis.

"My current adviser is great," she explained. "But my sophomore sociology professor was very hard on me. She told me I had no feel for the subject."

Heidi and I continued to explore her sensitivity to criticism over a number of sessions. Within two weeks of starting Lexapro, her panic attacks were all but gone, and she was able to taper off the Xanax. Every few weeks, however, Heidi would experience a tiny glimmer of panic symptoms. She was able to talk herself down when they occurred, but their timing—usually just before Heidi had to present her work to her adviser—provided us with an opportunity to better understand their meanings and origins.

After a month, Heidi's panic attacks went away completely, and we agreed to meet once a month. She graduated in May of that year but decided to remain on Lexapro for another year while working at her first job.

It may seem paradoxical, but Heidi was lucky that her anxiety symptoms were severe enough to demand immediate attention. Had they been less severe, she might have delayed getting proper treatment or, worse, tried to deal with them herself by using alcohol, pot, or prescription drugs.

Self-medicating is a big mistake. Unsupervised prescription drugs, pot, and alcohol *may* give some escape from the anxiety, but the relief will be short-lived. And, when the symptoms return, they will return with greater and greater ferocity. Once this cycle begins, it doesn't take long for the anxiety disorder to be overtaken by substance abuse. Then you have two problems, each aggravating the other and making the other harder to treat.

INSOMNIA

If, as Shakespeare asserts in *Macbeth*, sleep "knits up the raveled care of time," then insomnia leaves you totally unraveled. And it's a double whammy—because not only does insomnia make you fearful of whatever it is that's keeping you awake, it also makes you fearful of not being able to fall sleep. The fear of insomnia, in other words, *gives* you insomnia.

In college, insomnia—at least temporary insomnia—is virtually universal. Between noisy dorms and late-arriving roommates, heavy homework assignments, too much caffeine, and constant stress, college life is a recipe for delayed sleep. Just ask professors with 8:00 A.M. classes. And the usual rules of good sleep "hygiene"—dark, cool, quiet room; consistent bedtime; absence of stimulations like the Internet, TV, and socializing; getting under the covers only to sleep— are pretty much impossible. It's almost amazing that most college students, most of the time, are able to fall asleep and stay asleep once they finally try to do so.

Insomnia is *insomnia* only if you can't fall asleep or fall back to sleep within about half an hour of trying to do so. And it's only a problem if you have insomnia more than once or twice a week and it begins to affect your physical or mental well-being or your ability to function.

By this definition, of course, almost every college student will experience insomnia sooner or later. What to do?

First you have to figure out whether the insomnia is primary or secondary. It's secondary if it's caused by some other problem like depression or panic disorder or recurrent nightmares or drugs or alcohol or a medical illness. It's primary if it's caused by sleep apnea, restless leg syndrome, poor sleep hygiene, or the fear of insomnia itself—or if there is no apparent cause at all.

If the insomnia is secondary, then the solution is to deal with the underlying cause: treat the depression; reduce the alcohol, caffeine, and Adderall; get a flu shot before you get sick. If the insomnia is primary, it may have to be attacked directly. Very often you will need to see a doctor in order to figure out whether it's primary or secondary.

The most common form of primary insomnia, especially in college, is persistent difficulty falling asleep or poor-quality sleep for which there is no apparent cause. The problem is the insomnia itself and the anxiety it causes—and, of course, the rotten feeling it produces the following day—not some underlying psychiatric or medical disorder. If you have this garden variety form of insomnia, you've probably had trouble falling asleep during elementary and high school as well. The pain of being awake when everyone else is sleeping, the self-perpetuating fear of lying in bed worrying, and the dread that grows as the dark of night approaches will be all too familiar to you. And the cruel paradox—that you have no trouble napping during the day even though you can't fall asleep at night—only makes matters worse.

If you've tried the conventional recommendations for good sleep hygiene—consistent bedtime, favorable sleep environment, and disciplined sleep rituals—and *still* can't fall asleep, you're among the vast majority of insomniacs. The problem with sleep hygiene techniques is 1. they're hard to apply in the college or any real-life situation and 2. they rarely seem to work even if you're able to apply them.

So let's try to go back to basic principles and see if we can figure out a practical and effective way to combat insomnia.

First, what does it feel like to fall asleep naturally and how does that differ from what it feels like to have insomnia? Well, when you fall asleep naturally, your mind is filled with interesting *images*; when you have insomnia your mind is filled with perplexing and challenging *ideas*. When you fall asleep naturally, you indulge in pleasant *fantasies* and tell yourself wish-fulfilling *stories*; when you have insomnia, you have troubling *thoughts* and engage in circular *arguments* and debates or indulge in endless *recriminations*. When you fall asleep comfortably, your mind is at ease and already starting to *dream*; when you have insomnia, your mind is not at ease and continues to *cogitate*.

Now try to cast your memory back to childhood, before you ever had insomnia. Can you recall that wonderful wave of drowsiness that washed over you like a narcotic, sweeping you into blissful slumber before you even knew it? Can you recall giving yourself over to that druglike feeling without the slightest doubt or fear? Can you recall drinking in the sweetest sleep the way a parched traveler drinks in the purest water from an icy brook? Do you recall the beautiful images that floated across your consciousness just before you were carried off into the world of dreams? Do you recall trying to complete a story in your head before you fell asleep—a story in which you were the hero and wonderful things were happening to you? Do you remember that you couldn't help losing the thread of the narrative because you kept drifting off into slumber and because you never wanted your story to end?

Try to retain those memories from childhood, because we're going to use them very soon to help you relearn how to fall asleep.

But, first, what caused your insomnia? Falling asleep used to be so simple, so foolproof. What happened to make such a painful hash of it?

The answer is: life happened. Anxiety happened. Awareness of danger and death happened. Nightmares and scary stories and fear of the dark happened. Neurophysiology and overstimulation and sounds in the night happened. As you got older, homework and worries about school and conflicts with friends and regrets over mistakes happened. Most of all, the fear of unconsciousness—the fear of being defenseless while asleep—happened.

But whatever the cause—whether you feared being unconscious or just wanted more time to solve the problems of the day—sleep became the enemy. Instead of welcoming the urge to sleep, you fought it. And you won the fight.

Eventually the ability to resist sleep became automatic—so automatic, in fact, that now you can't fall asleep even when you want to. And, instead of lulling you into sweet unconsciousness, that once welcome wave of sleepiness makes you merely toss and turn.

Riding the Sleep Wave

The secret to overcoming primary insomnia is learning—actually relearning—how to ride the wave of sleepiness that came so naturally in early childhood. It involves remembering what the sleep wave felt like in the past before you had insomnia so you can recognize and ride it into sleep again in the present. If you can't remember your preinsomnia days, perhaps you can recall what the sleep wave felt like from more recent experiences such as when you were really, really sleep deprived or jet-lagged, spent a long physically taxing day outside, took an over-the-counter sleeping pill, or were back in your old bed at home after many months away.

Though only a metaphor, the sleep wave is a lovely and delicious experience. But it's short-lived. You have to catch it when it first sweeps toward you and ride it into peaceful slumber. If you miss the first sleep wave early in the night, it may be a long time before the next one comes along. Now that you've trained yourself to ignore or resist the sleep wave, you may have to pay closer attention to the signs that it's creeping toward you. You may find yourself denying the feeling of drowsiness or reacting to it with anxiety and fear. Despite wanting to overcome your insomnia, a part of you will still try to fight falling asleep. You'll get wrapped up in some stimulating or necessary activity (like surfing the Web) or begin trying to solve some interpersonal problem from today or tomorrow.

You may find it helpful to develop a bedtime ritual that allows you to shed the worries of the day and prepare yourself for the arrival of the sleep wave. (I notice that a vague feeling of dread clings to the phrase "prepare for the arrival of the sleep wave," as if I were saying "prepare for the arrival of the bogeyman.") One young woman I treated found it helpful to clear her mind before bed by writing in her diary; another unwound from the cares of the day by meditating.

It's important to be in bed, perhaps reading something pleasant but not too exciting, when the first ripples of sleepiness roll in so you can turn out the light and ride the crest of the wave into sleep. If you find yourself struggling to stay awake, try to think of the sleep wave not as a huge wall of water forcing you under but as an ocean swell gently lifting you up and setting you down. You need to remove the element of fear. You need to feel that sleep is your friend the way a balmy breeze is your friend or a loving hug is your friend. You need to be able to embrace the sleep wave and pleasantly drift on it, not fight it like an undertow.

But sometimes you can't make yourself relax enough to enjoy the feeling of weariness and let it drift you into restorative unconsciousness. Sometimes you *want* to sleep but *can't*—you can't turn off your mind or stop planning or worrying long enough to relax. Sometimes—like when you have an exam the next day—it's so urgent you sleep that the very urgency makes it hard to do so. Sometimes you want to sleep but also *don't* want to sleep. You know you're going to feel exhausted the next day, but *right now* you refuse to give in. So you lay there, wide awake, fretting about not being able to fall asleep but totally unable—or unwilling—to do so.

Sleep Medication

This is where sleeping pills come in. Sleeping pills are highly effective in helping insomniacs fall asleep or return to sleep if they awaken during the night. But sleeping pills—*all* sleeping pills—are a double-edged sword: if they succeed in helping you to fall and stay asleep, they may make you feel hung over the following morning. If you stay on them for an extended period of time, they tend to lose their efficacy, which means you have to raise the dose or change pills. And if you use them every night, it's easy to become dependent on them. (Remember, being dependent is different from being addicted, because there is no craving for sleeping pills, no drug-seeking behavior, and no using them to get high.) These caveats apply as much to over-the-counter drugs, like Benadryl (pure diphenhydramine), Tylenol PM (Tylenol plus diphenhydramine), and Advil PM (Advil plus diphenhydramine), as they do to prescription drugs like Ambien, Restoril, and Lunesta. Nevertheless, there are millions of people who take some kind of sedative medication every night for sleep without any apparent ill effects, except that eventually they can't sleep without it.

Here's the approach I take to treat insomnia when the person hasn't been able to consistently recognize and ride his sleep wave into natural sleep, where he can't practice good sleep hygiene, or where he needs occasional help falling or staying asleep. It is neither puritanical nor particularly original, and it's certainly not the last word.

1. I recommend that the person with insomnia cut out caffeine and alcohol, especially later in the day. Even small amounts of caffeine taken early in the morning can make it more difficult for some people to fall asleep at night. And because alcohol is a very short-acting sedative, it can cause you to wake up hyperalert after several hours of sleep, even if it helped you conk out at the beginning of the night.

2. Next, I will prescribe a benzodiazepine with an intermediate half-life, such as Restoril or Dalmane, to be taken thirty to sixty minutes before bedtime. I tend to prefer a benzodiazepine to drugs like Ambien because the benzos have more of an antianxiety effect, which is helpful in dealing with the worrying that causes and accompanies insomnia. If anxiety is a prominent feature of the insomnia, I may recommend a longer-lasting benzodiazepine like Valium or Klonopin. It may make sense to take these drugs earlier in the evening, rather than just before bedtime, to help you feel calmer and fall asleep more naturally and to minimize residual drowsiness upon awakening the next morning.

Ambien and Lunesta were marketed as less habit-forming than the benzodiazepines (the Valium drugs) and less likely to lose efficacy over time. I'm not convinced this putative advantage is really true. Ambien is just as likely to be used to get high as the benzos, has rare but disturbing side effects (like visual hallucinations and amnesia) that are uncommon in longer-acting benzos, and is nearly as likely to stop working effectively as the benzos. Nevertheless, I have no trouble prescribing Ambien or Lunesta if they are preferred or if anxiety is not a prominent feature of the insomnia. Many people do well on these medicines for months or years.

I think it's preferable to take sleeping pills at the beginning of the night, even if your problem is waking up in the middle of the night. Most sleeping pills will give you a hangover unless you have at least seven hours to sleep after taking them. Medicines that get out of your system quickly, like Sonata, low-dose Ativan, or Xanax, can be used for the occasional episode of insomnia that occurs in the middle of the night. But, if you're one of the large number of people who has "middle insomnia" virtually every night, it might be worth experimenting to see whether increasing the dose of your sleeping pill at bedtime works better than trying to decide at 4:00 A.M. whether or not to take a booster dose.

3. I avoid prescribing the very potent drugs like Seroquel or Zyprexa for insomnia except for very short periods of time when the person is agitated and other drugs have failed. These drugs are very

effective for insomnia, but their effects can last well into the next day and they often cause very rapid weight gain. Even absent these short-term problems, we have no idea what the long-term side effects of these relatively new drugs might be if taken over many months or years merely for sleep.

Some doctors prescribe low doses of older antidepressants, such as amitriptyline or trazodone, for chronic insomnia on the assumption that they are less habit-forming than conventional sleep medications. This class of medicines is less abusable than, say, Restoril or Ambien, but you can still become psychologically dependent on them. The antidepressants also have more (though generally mild) side effects, and don't always work as well, as the dedicated sleeping pills. Some patients also try melatonin and other natural sleep aids. Though benign, these sleep aids are less potent than conventional medications, yet still capable of producing dependence and side effects.

4. After the patient has begun sleeping well for a week or so, I encourage her to begin using the sleep medicine intermittently. Most people will do this on their own. With luck, the insomnia will become more sporadic and the medication can be used on an as-needed basis. Many students, however, will elect to wait until the end of the semester before trying to go off their sleep meds.

Final Thoughts on Insomnia

Some people sleep better when there's someone else in bed with them; some people sleep worse. Some people sleep better when they're at home with their families; some people sleep better when they're in their own places. Some people are disciplined about practicing good sleep hygiene—and still have trouble falling asleep without pills; some people do everything wrong and fall asleep as soon as their heads hits the pillow.

Sometimes you can arrange to be in the optimal circumstances for *you* to fall asleep; most of the time—especially if you're a college student—you can't. So insomnia, at least occasionally, is inevitable.

Here are a few final suggestions for dealing with insomnia:

1. Spend some time every day outside in the sunlight. Bright light helps set your biological clock to the correct diurnal cycle. Without adequate daytime exposure to light, many people will begin to feel drowsy during the day and hyperalert at night. (Just ask the students who are going to college in Maine or Michigan during the winter semester!)

Indoor lighting is generally not strong enough to signal your brain that it's daytime. The 10,000 Lux lights that are used for treating seasonal affective disorder (SAD) are strong enough to entrain your sleep-wake cycle. If you are sleepy during the day and wide awake at night, try resetting your internal clock by going outside or getting a light box.

The most common way your sleep-wake cycle will get out of sync with the day-night cycle is to have trouble waking up before 10:00 A.M. and trouble falling asleep before midnight or even 2:00 A.M. If you have this "phase-shift" disorder, you'll find that you don't wake up in the morning spontaneously, that you often sleep through your alarm and are chronically late, that you tend to sleep even later on weekends when you have no early appointments, that you're groggy, irritable, and out of sorts until noon, that your mental acuity is diminished, and that you're drowsy in the afternoon but wide awake at bedtime. In order to correct this phase shift, you need to move your wake-up time *very gradually* forward by getting up fifteen to thirty minutes earlier in the morning and exposing yourself to bright daylight or a light box for the first half hour after rising.

If you're used to getting up at 10:00 A.M., start by going outside for a half-hour walk at 10:00 A.M. If there is no bright light outside because of the season or the weather, get a light box and sit eighteen inches from it for half an hour on waking. Eventually, your brain will be trained to signal the need for sleep (by sending you a sleep wave) approximately eight hours before the expected light exposure in the morning. Every few days, or longer if needed, you should push your wake-up time—and light exposure—fifteen to thirty minutes earlier. By doing this, you will gradually synchronize your sleep-wake cycle to the local day-night cycle. You should be able to wake up and go to sleep spontaneously at the appropriate times and feel rested and alert during the day.

You can apply the same principle (exposing yourself to morning sunlight) when you're studying abroad to help get over jet lag.

2. Dorms and apartments—with students coming and going, tapping on their keyboards, listening to music, talking, and partying at all hours—are noisy. If the noise is keeping you awake, try a white-noise maker. (No, a white-noise maker is not a device for generating hillbilly music. It's a machine that generates a soothing background noise that covers—and thus muffles—a range of frequencies.) You can experiment with a noisy electric fan before buying a white-noise machine. If you find it soothing (and your roommate doesn't hate it), you can buy a dedicated device that, unlike a fan, won't blow cold air on you all winter.

Some white-noise makers electronically simulate the sound of rain, the ocean, or the jungle at night. These sounds are never accurate and can become irritating. A simple device with a small fan inside a plastic cylinder that vents through tiny holes in the side generates a uniform background sound and is more soothing. You can even use it to blot out noise when you're trying to study during the day—although I wouldn't bring it to the library.

3. Try to imagine that you're sleeping in the arms of or next to someone you love. Imagine this person is soothing you (or arousing you if that makes you drowsy). And imagine that he or she is awake when you are and falls asleep when you do. Don't let this fantasy make you feel depressed or lonely. And don't feel sheepish about having to resort to this fantasy in order to feel safe and calm enough to fall asleep. One day there may be someone who sleeps with you every night. And, after you adjust to sharing your bed with this person you love, you *will* sleep better—just like in your fantasy. In the meantime, you might also try your blankie or a teddy bear.

Drugs and Alcohol

COLLEGE STUDENTS ARE USING DRUGS more than in the past; college drug use is declining. Alcohol abuse is rampant on college campuses; the alcohol problem in college is less than commonly assumed. Alcohol has become the drug of choice for college students; prescription drug use is increasing. Every new study on substance use and abuse among college students says something a little different, sometimes even contradictory. Suffice it to say: substance abuse in general, and alcohol abuse in particular, is a problem on college campuses.

Substance abuse comes in two flavors: addiction and bingeing. Addiction receives more attention because it's more serious and more difficult to treat. It involves habitual use, craving, withdrawal symptoms, and dose escalation to achieve the desired effect. Addicts are hooked on their drug, and they will devote time and resources to get it. Addiction is what wrecks people's lives and sends them to rehab.

But bingeing is a bigger problem on college campuses than full-blown addiction—because it doesn't necessarily *seem* like a problem.

If you're a college student, you typically binge on drugs, and especially alcohol, at parties with friends. The fact that you're not doing it alone, that you're doing it only once or twice a week, and that a lot of other people at the party are drinking excessively too makes bingeing seem normal. No, *better* than normal: getting hammered on weekends seems like the quintessence of what it means to be in college. The drunken lacrosse player puking in the street or the dolled-up sorority girl tripping on her high heels as she descends the stairs to the frat house is what you think of when you think of having fun. Beer pong is as much a part of your vision of college life as ivy-covered buildings and all-nighters in the library. You smile when you see boisterous students staggering home from the pub or getting belligerent at a tailgating party. Getting drunk or stoned with friends is how you bond. It's part of your identity as a college student.

Most of the time the only consequences of a weekend binge are a bad hangover, lost items of clothing, and a wasted study day. But sometimes the consequences are more serious: a drug overdose, alcohol poisoning, date rape, an arrest for DUI, broken bones, or a visit to the emergency room. Because it entails excess rather than moderation, bingeing is not only dangerous in itself but dangerous also because it increases the risk of addiction. True, the slope from bingeing to addiction may not be as slippery as the public service announcements on television would have you believe. But every year a few thousand students nationwide manage to slide down it.

The reasons for abuse are a little different for each substance, but they have several things in common: they get you high—and it's fun to get high; they break down inhibitions, including sexual inhibitions; they facilitate socializing and partying; they dispel both anxiety *and* boredom; they're cool and make you feel part of the gang; and they're only a problem if you use them excessively, which, you tell yourself, is a problem that applies only to other people (although, for many college students, using drugs excessively is precisely the point of using them in the first place). Finally, there are few people *dis*couraging you—and many people *en*couraging you—to use drugs in college.

Here are some of the ways college students use and abuse alcohol and drugs and rationalize doing so:

Alcohol is readily available and, depending on the drinking age, quasi-legal. It is the elixir of the frat party and the lubricant of dining and dating. True, a relatively small number of you will die every year of alcohol poisoning, car accidents, and injuries. And many of you will do stupid and dangerous things while drunk. But most of you will drink with impunity. Suffering only minor consequences leads to the erroneous belief that bad things that *could* happen *won't* happen—at least not to you—because you "know your limit" and you're able to stick to your limit even after a few drinks.

Pot is the catalyst for late-night bull sessions, the appreciation of music and pop culture, and the escape from work. You can use pot as a treatment for anxiety or insomnia. And it's a great excuse for skipping classes.

Cocaine feels good and helps you study—unless you get addicted to it (which, of course, can't happen to you, since you have it under control). Once you're addicted to cocaine, you *certainly* have drug cravings and *may* have depression, nasal damage, heart attacks, strokes, or seizures.

Prescription drugs—opiates, sedatives, and stimulants—are abused not only because they get you high but also because they help you pull all-nighters and stay focused, fall asleep when you're overstimulated, and control your appetite. All these drugs have dangerous side effects and are highly addictive (though, naturally, not for you).

I apologize for the sarcasm, but every student I've seen who has gotten into trouble with drugs (including alcohol) started out convinced that he wouldn't get into trouble with drugs. No one started using drugs in order to get hooked; she started using drugs in order to get high with friends. After awhile, however, getting high more or less became the *basis* of friendships.

I realize, too, that most of you will experiment with drugs, especially mainstream drugs like alcohol, pot—even coke and hallucinogens—without becoming addicted. You'll be able to stop before your use gets out of control—at least that's what you hope. You'll be aware of the dangers of drugs and alcohol, try them anyway, and stop before they've become a problem. Given the reality that only a minority of college students end up damaged by drugs, my sarcasm—like government warnings, public service ads, and the rules found in every college's student handbook—will seem ridiculous. Unfortunately, psychoactive substances don't respect good intentions, strong willpower, the resilience of youth, or sophisticated knowledge. They claim their victims from among the smart, healthy, and well informed as easily as among the limited, needy, and ignorant.

You should know that, as a college student, you are more vulnerable to drug abuse because you feel more *invulnerable*. And you're also more vulnerable because you're more vulnerable. Why? Because you're coping with stresses that are peculiar to college—homesickness, work pressure, peer pressure, new independence, social anxiety, and self-doubt—in unfamiliar surroundings and without the immediate support of home and family.

Drug *abuse* (including alcohol abuse) always begins as drug *use*. And sometimes it begins as a way to self-medicate psychological problems. Sedating drugs, like alcohol, pot, Valium, Klonopin, Xanax, and Ambien, are used to self-treat anxiety and insomnia. Stimulant drugs, like cocaine, Ritalin, Dexedrine, and Adderall, are used to self-treat depression and difficulties concentrating and studying. Stimulants also help keep you alert during all-nighters and reinforce the tyranny of having to be thin by giving students with eating disorders a tool for controlling their appetites. (Students with eating disorders should note, however, that the stimulants are a poor way to control appetite: they often lose efficacy and they weaken healthier controls on dietary intake.) Opiates, like codeine, oxycodone, and hydrocodone are used to self-treat anxiety and depression as well as to get high.

When you use drugs to "treat" problems, you are really *misusing* them—and you know it. The drugs have either been obtained from another student, or, if obtained from your doctor, are not being used in the doses, or for the reasons, prescribed.

Unfortunately, by the time substance *use* has migrated across the vague and porous border into *abuse*, you will be inclined (like most people) to deny you have a problem, rationalize your use, or overestimate your ability to control it. You will be unable to see a way out, feel too ashamed to tell your parents and get expert help, or, finally (in desperation), profess not to care. This is regrettable, because—once acknowledged and treated—drug problems are highly (no pun intended) treatable.

Most colleges have programs to help students with drug and alcohol problems. Unfortunately, many college students are too embarrassed to make use of them. If you're one of these embarrassed people or the on-campus programs are not rigorous enough for you, get a referral to a psychiatrist or counselor in the community or back home who deals with substance abuse and with whom you feel comfortable.

If there is no substance abuse program or therapist in your college community—and even if there is—it might also be helpful to attend meetings of Alcoholics Anonymous or Narcotics Anonymous. Every community has at least one AA meeting (and often an NA meeting). If there's no NA chapter, you should go to AA. Many branches of AA will accept people whose principal problem isn't alcohol and all AA meetings can help you locate a twelve-step program that does deal with your problem.

I know what you're thinking. *I don't need outside help—and I certainly don't need AA. AA is for drunks. Alcohol isn't my drug of choice. AA is too religious. And AA is too predicated on "sharing" and groupthink.* You're thinking: *I'm not really alcoholic, religiosity irritates me, and I hate groups—I'll just stop drinking!*

Maybe you will succeed in overcoming your alcoholism or drug abuse by moderation or temporary abstinence. Some people do. But many do not. They relapse over and over again. Since you don't want to squander your opportunity to continue in college by flunking out, being kicked out, or developing an illness, you should get help. And you should stick with it beyond the first few visits. Because of the shame, denial, and rationalization associated with substance abuse, you will want to disparage the treatment or talk yourself out of it. You will look for all the inherent contradictions, the uncomfortable rituals and the scientific loopholes in the treatment, and use them to wriggle out of going. You'll go back to trying to limit your drug or alcohol use on your own—and you'll probably fail.

Here's what I know about AA and other twelve-step programs: they work. People who stick with them for one year show more improvement in their lives than almost any other kinds of patients I treat. People who go to AA with an open mind are pleased to discover that the other people in AA are often just like them—they are all ages and come from every socioeconomic and educational background. People who go to AA are relieved to discover that the other people in AA have a range of religious beliefs and that many have no formal religious beliefs at all. And they are surprised to discover that AA is highly pro-social: contrary to expectations, AA doesn't foster self-pity and narcissism but does foster accountability, humility, and service to others. And, believe it or not, despite their seriousness of purpose, AA meetings are enjoyable. There's usually a lot of humor, and you always leave a meeting having learned something important—about life and about yourself—and feeling better.

If the first few meetings you go to don't seem to be a good fit, try other meetings until you find one where you feel comfortable with the culture and the people. You should feel accepted, you should feel inspired, and you should feel that you belong. Most AA members will move around a little before they find their "home group" and a simpatico sponsor.

AA isn't for everyone. Not everyone needs it and not everyone likes it. But, before you decide whether it is or isn't for you, check it out. Look up a beginner's meeting or an open meeting online, or ask someone who attends AA which meeting she recommends. Then go. Go a few times. And go with an open mind.

Body Image, Eating Disorders and Self-harm

BODY IMAGE

We live in a tyranny. It is a tyranny enforced by strict codes of behavior, unrelenting propaganda in the media, and insidious peer pressure. It is a tyranny built on a single totalitarian idea so all encompassing and seductive that even those who know better have trouble resisting it. The pernicious idea on which this tyranny is based is that *thinness equals beauty*. We are indoctrinated in this totalitarian equation at every waking moment of our lives, from childhood through old age, not by the government but by ourselves. It infects family life, school life, work life, friendship, and, of course, romance.

Like many cultural phenomena, thinness is a feminist issue: Though both sexes are affected by the quest to achieve thinness, women suffer from it more than men. There is hardly a female anywhere in the first world who is unconcerned about her weight. (I say "female," not "woman," because the tyranny of thinness affects all age groups from prepubescent girls to elderly women.)

In truth, almost no one of either sex is immune. Even though notions of beauty are more elastic for males than for females, men are not immune from the tyranny of thinness. Like their female counterparts, most male actors and models work hard—sometimes too hard—at being muscular, which puts pressure on other young men to follow suit. And most men, like most women, feel obligated to watch their weight in order to be attractive. Not surprisingly, more and more young men are developing eating disorders, which often go unrecognized until they are quite severe.

If thinness equals beauty, then parents will want their children to be thin (if only to avoid the problems of being obese), girls will want to be thin and to associate with other girls who are thin, boys will find thin girls more attractive, employers will favor thin employees, and so forth. Thinness will come to be associated with other desirable traits—self-discipline, greater education, higher social class, superior genes, and better health—the thinner the better.

The problem is that most young women are not naturally thin. After puberty most young women are rounded. They're zaftig, nubile, womanly. This used to be considered a good thing. It still is a good thing. It signifies fecundity and health. It is also beautiful. But you'll have a hard time trying to convince a young woman living under the tyranny of thinness that this is so. You could try to radicalize her by exposing her to revolutionary ideas like "love your body as it is" or "pursue healthy nutrition" or " base self-esteem on accomplishment and inner beauty." But she will quote back to you the banal slogans and approving pictorials of *Us* magazine and *ET*, where the smiling celebrities who've been "cured" of their eating disorders are still ridiculously thin.

EATING DISORDERS

Now, in theory, college campuses ought to be a place where the tyranny of thinness can be challenged. The culture of the university is antiauthoritarian. College students and faculty tend to be more resistant to conventional ideas, especially "bourgeois" ideas of gender identity, beauty, and virtue. And college is the place where it's safer than in the outside world to experiment with alternative ways of thinking and living. It's a place where you're supposed to discover who you are and to be yourself.

In practice, however, college campuses are not immune from the pervasive influences of the surrounding culture. And because they are also places where young people compete for recognition and romantic partners, they exert tremendous social pressure to conform to the prevailing notion of what's attractive. In that context, bucking the tyranny of thinness can seem like a risky strategy. Some of you will have the robust self-esteem, personal courage, or innate rebelliousness to do so or will find a social milieu in which you're able to find acceptance regardless of your weight. Most of you will submit to the harsh equation that thinness equals beauty and do your best to keep your weight in check. More than a few of you, unfortunately, will strive for extreme thinness by starving yourselves, purging, or using amphetamines. You'll believe that you're failing to meet the harsh standards imposed by the tyranny of thinness. In reality, you will be falling ill from your delusion.

Because you believe your problem is not too much thinness but too little, trying to "deprogram you" from years of indoctrination about the desirability of extreme thinness is often futile. The better course of action is to assure your safety (by making sure you don't die of starvation or malnutrition) and treat the psychological underpinnings of your eating disorder (the quirks that made you *particularly* susceptible to the tyranny of thinness).

Assuring your physical health usually involves collaboration between a psychiatrist, nutritionist, and internist. It *always* involves making sure you are adequately nourished with amino acids, electrolytes, vitamins, etc. It *often* involves trying to help you accept a target of 90 percent of your ideal body weight.

Working on your psychological health is more complicated. Issues of control over yourself and others, competition with siblings and peers, self-acceptance and the acceptance of limits and imperfections, fears of growing up and of sexuality can all be involved in making you vulnerable to an eating disorder. Depression and anxiety increase the risk. Very often there is also a triggering event that planted the eating disorder seed on the fertile soil of your particular psyche. The seed might be an incident in which you felt insulted or complimented about your weight, a competitive defeat or victory involving a sibling or friend, a cry for your parents' attention, or any number of things. It might even be something you "caught," like the flu, from someone else with an eating disorder—a peer or a celebrity. Because the triggering event often contains within it both the cause and the cure of your disordered eating, looking at it closely in therapy can be very productive.

Treatment for eating disorders involves individual psychotherapy and sometimes family and/or group therapy as well. The problem, of course, is that, because of your mortal dread of being persuaded or forced to gain weight, you'll avoid treatment in the first place and resist it once you're in. Unlike depressed patients who feel *worse* as they get sicker, you may feel *better*—more powerful and more in control—as you get sicker. As a result, the impetus for seeking treatment may come from someone else—from your therapist, your family doctor, or, most likely, from your parents.

If you're in college away from home, however, it may be one of your friends who first notices that you have an eating disorder. And if you *are* that friend—or a dean, an athletic coach, a boyfriend or a girlfriend—what should you do? If you feel close to your anorexic or bulimic friend, or trusted by her as a mentor, you can try to respectfully and supportively express your concern. If her eating behaviors are making it hard for you to be comfortable with her, you can lovingly tell her so. But, if you're unable or unwilling to confront her directly, or she seems to be getting worse and worse, you should contact her parents and leave it to them to deal with her.

Unfortunately, it can take some time before even parents or doctors are able to recognize that a college student has an eating disorder. They have to overcome their own conditioning that thinness is desirable. And because their child or patient may have started out "chubby" and "needed to lose some weight," it may even look at first as though she is dieting appropriately. Many anorexics are fond of cooking for others and will appear to be eating their meals when they're really just moving food around on their plates. And, because they binge and purge in secret and may not even appear to be underweight, most bulimics will fly beneath the radar until someone finally notices that their behavior around meals is suspicious.

The subtle clues that something is wrong with your eating behavior (or your child's eating behavior) include changes in behavior at mealtime, idiosyncratic diets and fastidiousness about caloric intake, eating at odd times, including late at night, secretly stashing and bingeing on junk food, compulsive exercising, general guardedness and irritability, and defensiveness when the topic of eating behavior is raised. The obvious clues that something is wrong with your eating behavior are purging (self-induced diarrhea or vomiting) or significant weight loss.

But even before eating behavior becomes aberrant and any weight has been lost, the future anorexic or bulimic begins to view food and her body as the enemy. Every mouthful is seen as a defeat—a giving in to bodily urges—and every feeling of fullness is experienced as unpleasant bloating. If you find yourself pinching a fold of skin and angrily telling yourself that you're disgusting, you're setting the stage for anorexia (unless it only happens when you're premenstrual). If you feel elated after you regurgitate a meal, you're at risk of becoming addicted to the "high" of purging.

Strictly speaking, anorexia nervosa requires weight loss that drops you below 85 percent of your ideal body weight. But since the "disorder" is already underway well before you've lost that much weight, it's better to seek professional consultation when you're "merely" obsessing about your weight and eating or dieting compulsively. The same applies if you're bingeing and vomiting or using laxatives or diuretics. Purging can cause damage to your teeth and digestive tract as well as very serious nutritional and electrolyte imbalances.

More common than anorexia and bulimia is "binge-eating disorder," which may or may not result in weight gain and may or may not lead to purging (i.e., to bulimia). Binge eating is very disturbing because it raises the specter of weight gain and makes you feel out of control. You will probably try to deal with it by skipping meals, which only makes you more ravenous and more likely to binge later on, or by restricting the *size* of your meals, which only leads to bingeing on junk. There are a variety of pragmatic and effective treatments for binge eating disorder so, again, seek professional help.

All eating disorders are easiest to treat when treated early. So don't dismiss your suspicion that there is something wrong or wait until you're absolutely sure you have an eating disorder. Once you have the suspicion that you have anorexia, bulimia, or binge eating, get advice from a doctor with expertise in eating disorders.

As with depression, there are milder forms of eating disorders. These are so prevalent and unremarkable that they seem almost normal.

If you're a typical student with a mild eating disorder, you're probably a freshman or sophomore who is perfectionistic about your schoolwork, self-critical about your conduct with friends, and obsessed with your weight. Though you know better, you can't resist comparing yourself with other young women on campus (except that you only compare yourself with women who are very, very thin.)

Every now and then you'll have a little freak-out triggered by something trivial. Here's an example. You and your roommate (who is invariably petite and always gets her work done on time) decide to take a break from studying to watch TV and order a pizza. When the pizza comes, she has one or two slices, eating only the cheese and toppings, sips her Diet Coke until the program is over, then says good-bye and goes back to writing her essay. You finish the rest of the pizza, crust and all, then watch a dumb reality show. By the time you've watched several more hours of television (and possibly finished a bag of cookies), your roommate has completed her essay and is heading for the gym. The minute she shuts the door, you call your mother and pick a fight:

"I'm so depressed, mom. I feel like killing myself!"
"Why? What's the matter, sweetheart?"
"I'm a fat loser!"

"No you're not, darling. You're a beautiful young woman."

"Don't humor me. I'm fat and I'm probably going to flunk out."

(*Starting to get worried*) "Why do you say that? Aren't you doing your work?"

"How can you ask me that? It's none of your business. I don't need you putting pressure on me."

"Are you getting your period? You always feel overwhelmed before your period. Maybe that's why you're feeling fat. Everyone binges and feels bloated around their period."

"No!" (*Yes.*) "It's just too hard for me here. I'm overwhelmed."

After an hour on the phone . . .

"You're not helping me, Mom. I told you, I'm a fat, stupid pig!"

"I'm doing my best, dear. Why don't you just take a little break and start your work after you've calmed down."

"Oh, Mom, you just don't get it!"

Because you're too embarrassed (or too much in denial) to tell her what's *really* depressing you—that you've "indulged" yourself by bingeing and watching TV instead of doing your schoolwork and that you've "betrayed" your friendship with your roommate by resenting her self-discipline—*your mother* hangs up feeling worried sick and *you* hang up feeling guilty and misunderstood. The next day, when your period has started and you're feeling better, you punish your mother further by "forgetting" to call her back with a reassuring update.

SELF-HARM

There are a whole bunch of self-injurious behaviors that young people pick up from their friends or from the cultural zeitgeist. These include the use of vomiting, laxatives, stimulants, and idiosyncratic diets to control weight; self-cutting and burning to deal with intense emotions, numbness, or boredom; and binge drinking and drug abuse to facilitate socialization. As with contagious diseases, some people are more resistant to these disorders and some are more susceptible.

In saying that these behaviors can be acquired by seeing other people do them, or even by reading about them or seeing them depicted on the screen, I'm in no way implying that they are trivial or *merely* willful. Self-harm has many causes and reflects real pain. (Including the *absence* of pain, such as when cutting or burning is used to pierce emotional numbness.) What I am saying is that, like other bad habits, these maladies *begin* as voluntary behaviors and that most of you, had you never seen or heard about them—from movies, books, or your friends—would probably *not* have come up with them on your own. In other words, had purging and cutting not been culturally available, you might have "chosen" some other response to psychic pain or numbness. Once having been chosen, however, self-injurious behaviors have a way of becoming self-perpetuating and habitual.

Stopping bad habits is hard. Stopping *self-destructive* bad habits is especially hard because popular culture has endowed suffering with a perverse glamour. We have made self-inflicted misery chic. Watching your own blood ooze from a cut you made yourself, burning your thigh with a cigarette, vomiting in a restaurant bathroom after a meal, letting yourself look like a derelict—all the sad and sordid acts associated with the "dark side"—are in reality little more than pop culture clichés. They equate misery with creativity, self-inflicted pain with martyrdom, and self-indulgence with nobility. Their sources are the literature of tragedy at its least imaginative—vampire cults, drug-martyred musicians and actors, mental asylum memoirs, and too-rich-for-their-own-good celebrity profiles. They borrow from the language of the street, but have no meaning beyond the self. Sadly, they are utterly derivative and unoriginal.

But they don't seem that way when you're young. They seem romantic. They feed upon the desire to make your life extraordinary, to be greater than it currently is. You want your life to be filled with passion and creativity. You want your pain to have meaning—something grander than the run-of-the-mill angst of the typical college student. You want your pain to be cinematic. But by dramatizing your angst and your uniqueness in this conventional way—by inflicting injury on yourself—you're not elevating it, you're diminishing it. By hyping it, you're saying that your pain is too trivial to be taken seriously on its own merits. You're saying it can't be spoken about in a reasonable way to a sympathetic listener; it has to be performed on a stark stage for an (imaginary) audience. You're paying a big price for the banality of our films and television.

But regardless of how these self-injurious behaviors began, they quickly take on a life of their own. They cease to become an *expression* of pain and become a self-perpetuating *source* of pain. As with drugs, the "cure" for the illness becomes the illness. Cutting and purging break away from their root causes and become very bad habits or even addictions.

Knowing that self-injurious behaviors are culturally determined and can quickly become habitual increases the importance of prevention. Here are some suggestions for preemption: 1. Reduce your exposure to people who are practicing self-damaging behaviors, especially if they—the people as well as the behaviors—seem appealing. 2. Improve your choice of movies and books. Be skeptical of "memoirs" that glamorize booze, drugs, self-degradation, and risk taking by turning them into "art." 3. If you've experimented with cutting or purging, stop immediately before those behaviors become habitual. 4. Better yet, think of them as disgusting addictions and avoid starting them in the first place.

Here's what we know so far about self-harming behaviors: they begin in deep emotions like loneliness, self-doubt, and sadness or in the absence of deep emotions like the "feelings" of emptiness, numbness, and boredom. Because "ordinary" outlets, like dialogue or healthy action, seem either too paltry or too difficult to employ, these emotions get expressed through behaviors, such as purging, cutting, and reckless drug use, that have been made "appealing" by popular culture. After awhile, these behaviors become hard-to-break habits.

But there is one additional aspect of these self-harming behaviors that we need to understand, because understanding it helps to explain why these behaviors are so appealing to young people on the cusp of adulthood: *all these self-injurious behaviors are a form of communica-*

tion. They are a communication to your *self.* (*I'm lonely, angry, sad, and overwhelmed. I don't know how to help myself and am too ashamed to ask for help directly.*) And they are a communication to the outside *world.* (*Help me! Save me from myself!*)

You may hate yourself, your parents, and the world; you may want to wallow in misery or be released from the boring and the mundane; you may even feel as though there is no purpose or meaning to life. But beneath all this unhappiness and nihilism there is a powerful hope—a hope you should grab onto and nourish—that you can still be rescued and redeemed. Beneath your existential angst and your loss of faith there is still a deep and abiding belief in the redemptive power of love.

To put it in concrete terms: when you hurt yourself, you hope that someone will love you enough to try to stop you. Consciously, that someone may be your ex-boyfriend, the girl who dumped you, or your best friend. But unconsciously, at the deepest level, that someone is your mother or your father. When you cut yourself or burn yourself or willfully wreck your life, one of the things you're saying is

Look, Mom and Dad. Look what's happened to your beloved child. Look what's become of the child you cherished and whose promise and potential we all rejoiced in. Look how low he's sunk. Look how miserable she's made herself. Why didn't you notice? Why didn't you stop me from hurting myself? Why don't you stop me from hurting myself? Why won't you pick me up and hug me and put a bandage on my scraped knee like you did when I was a child. Why won't you do the impossible? Why won't you make it all better?

There are two problems with expressing yourself this way (apart from its riskiness). One is that your parents might not be as hip to the cultural meaning of your acting out as you might hope. Instead of seeing your self-damaging behavior as a cry for help, they could misinterpret it as an act of rebellion—as an attack on them and their way of life. It's an easy mistake to make. And, in their understandable hurt and confusion, they might react with anger instead of encouragement and with rejection instead of support. If that were to happen—and it often does—your cry for help would go unheard. Your desperation would increase. And your urge to act out would get stronger and harder to stop.

The other problem with acting out instead of verbalizing your feelings is that it prevents you from facing the real issue—namely, that your parents *can't* make everything all right, even if they want to. And the reason they can't make everything all right—and maybe even shouldn't—is that you're on the cusp of adulthood, and, increasingly, your happiness is up to you. Your parents can *help* you with your problems. They can share their wisdom with you and give you their support. But they can't make your life productive and fulfilling. Only you can.

Recognizing that your fate is in your own hands is the key epiphany of adulthood. It's scary, but it's also liberating, because it means that you and no one else controls your destiny.

As a college student, your task is to begin to come to grips with this new reality—to see it not as a tragedy but as an opportunity. Your task is to overcome your fear and despair, to realign your relationship with your parents to reflect your growing independence and autonomy, and to develop the attitudes and skills you need to cope with and thrive in the adult world.

MEDICAL LEAVES OF ABSENCE

Sometimes it's prudent to take a leave of absence from school before your health deteriorates further or your academic record is blighted by poor performance. Leaves of absence on medical grounds have advantages and disadvantages over voluntary withdrawals. Because each college has different rules governing leaves, you should check your student handbook and consult with a dean and your parents before deciding to take a medical leave.

In general, medical leaves require the support of a doctor at the beginning and documentation of fitness to return at the end. They may also have minimum lengths of time, varying from one semester to one year, that have to be completed before you're eligible to return. Depending on the problem, you may have to show that you've successfully completed some sort of work or schooling while you've been on leave and, in many cases, will be continuing treatment once you're back in college. Voluntary withdrawals, where available, may have fewer requirements but can usually be taken only once.

There is no shame in taking a medical leave or voluntary withdrawal. Many students have availed themselves of the opportunity to take a break and returned to school healthier, more mature, and better able to take advantage of all that college has to offer.

Final Thoughts

Shame is the single biggest impediment to dealing with problems. Shame leads to avoidance. Shame leads to exaggeration of the problem in your own mind.

So let's deal with shame first.

Everyone confronts psychological problems sometime during his life. Nobody is exempt. Wealth, beauty, intelligence, a happy childhood, a good education, good parenting, good values, and good genes: none of these things can absolutely protect you against psychological problems. If you've been lucky up till now—congratulations. If you're having a problem for the first time—welcome.

The only reason you feel ashamed about having psychological problems is because you imagine—wrongly—that no one else is having problems or, more likely, because you imagine—again wrongly—that no one else *like you* is having problems. People like you—strong, smart, successful people—don't have problems. Only weak, limited, inept people do. Wrong! Having psychological problems doesn't mean you're abnormal; it means you're normal. It might even mean you're *better* than normal. It might mean you're more sensitive, more self-aware, and harder on yourself than your friends who seem to be sailing smoothly through.

To gain some perspective on how commonplace, and how routine, psychological problems are in college, let's briefly review some statistics:

Every semester since 1998, the American College Health Association surveys students at public and private universities, large and small, to determine the state of their health. They sample everyone from freshmen to doctoral students, and they cover every health issue from allergies to anorexia, from sinus infections to substance abuse.

I'll limit my focus to the problem of depression, which, because it is often a final common pathway for other difficulties—academic, social, psychological, and medical—is a reasonable proxy for significant distress.

In the spring of 2008, among a representative sample of 80,121 students, the American College Health Association survey found the following: at least once during the past school year, 93.7 percent of students reported "feeling overwhelmed by all they had to do," 91.8 percent reported "feeling exhausted (not from physical activity)," 78.7 percent reported "feeling very sad," 62.1 percent reported feeling "things were hopeless," and 43 percent reported "feeling so depressed it was difficult to function." Sadly, 9 percent "seriously considered attempting suicide" and 1.3 percent made an actual attempt.[1]

These depression data are remarkable. They say that nine out of ten university students will feel overwhelmed, mentally exhausted, or very sad at some point during the school year, and six out of ten will feel hopeless.

Feeling hopeless is no small thing. It is more than "ordinary unhappiness," which, according to Freud, is man's normal state. Hope-

1. American College Health Association, American College Health Association–National College Health Assessment (ACHA-NCHA) Reference Group Executive Summary, Spring 2008 (Baltimore: American College Health Association, 2008).

lessness is the state of having reached the limit of your ability to cope—or *believing* you've reached the limit of your ability to cope, which, luckily, is not quite the same thing. Sixty-two percent of students in the ACHA-NCHA Spring 2008 survey say they felt hopeless at least once during the school year. And that figure is just for one year. Over the four or five years most people spend in college, I think it's safe to assume that the cumulative numbers would be even higher.

Of course, not everyone who reports symptoms of depression will necessarily meet strict criteria for clinical depression. Even so, 14.9 percent of the students surveyed report having been "diagnosed with depression" at some time and, within this group, 32 percent report having been diagnosed with depression during the last school year. Of those with a history of clinical depression, 24.5 percent are "currently in therapy for depression" and 35.6 percent are "currently taking medication for depression."

I know there will be some of you—the hard cases—who will still feel ashamed of having a problem. It won't matter to you whether 10 percent or 90 percent of students experience emotional difficulties; it won't be OK for *you* to experience them. You will want to be part of that privileged group, however large or small, that is currently problem free. You have never wanted to be part of the masses anyway and you refuse to accept that you can't rise above your difficulties.

I respect your stoicism and self-reliance. I don't think that every problem needs to be professionally treated or that every hardship should be considered a disorder. Overcoming adversity, meeting challenges, coping with painful emotions: these are the stuff of life. I am not an advocate for the culture of therapy. I believe that people have a surprising amount of resilience and a great number of personal resources for dealing with adversity. I would never want to undermine those strengths by minimizing or pathologizing them.

So perhaps you're right. Perhaps you *can* tough it out. Maybe your problems really *are* no big deal and will somehow go away. And yet there is the thorny issue of shame. Shame makes you want to look away from a problem. It makes you feel small and weak and inadequate simply because you're flawed. And shame is a bigger problem for college students than for older adults because you don't yet have the worldly experience to know that problems are universal and that acknowledging them is a sign not of weakness but of strength.

College students also feel that they're in a fishbowl. You imagine that you're being watched by your classmates and teachers, your parents and their friends, your relatives, your girlfriends, boyfriends, and eventual employers—all of whom are expecting you to succeed brilliantly (or, in the case of rivals, secretly hoping for you to fail ignominiously). Even if this were true, which it may be to some degree, the people who really matter will be rooting for you and will understand that everybody flounders sometime or other. Your parents will come to grips with their own anxieties and disappointments—and your relationship with them will deepen because it will be more real. More important, since college is the stage in which you begin to develop independence, it will be a good time to begin to care less about what others think of you and to care more about your own concerns.

So, in short, if you're feeling depressed, overwhelmed, anxious, are floundering academically or socially, you're in good company—a vast company—and you now know what's it's like to be human. The only question is whether or not you can deal with your shame well enough to begin *working* on your problem. If the answer is yes, I hope this little book helps you do so.

If the answer is no—if you want to wait until you've hit a brick wall and you're *forced* to deal with the problem—fair enough. It's human nature to avoid difficult problems until you have no choice. But, when you reach that point, don't give up. The genius of the American education system is that there is always a second or third (or fourth) chance to make a new start. If you have to work for a few years and reenter college as a mature student, through general studies or by attending part-time, there is no shame in that. People mature at different ages. Not everyone is ready for college at eighteen. There are many, many students who, having floundered on their first or second attempt at college, triumphed on their third or fourth—and were better for it. We're all in too big a hurry anyway. What's the rush? By the time you're thirty, no one is going to know or care whether you took four years or eight years to graduate college—and they're not really going to care whether it was from Stanford or State.

One thing that's helpful regardless of what you chose to do is to try, if you can, to keep your sense of humor. Humor is how shame relieves itself. (I know it's a bad pun but that's precisely why it's appropriate!) Why do you think we laugh at the embarrassing screwups of characters on sitcoms? Why are the sick, politically incorrect jests of *South Park* and the hapless, self-important antics of Will Ferrell and Bernie Mac funny? Why do sex jokes and fart jokes still crack us up? Why are scenes of someone tracking dog poop into her house or meeting his girlfriend with his fly undone more hilarious than clever puns and witty repartee? Why do the embarrassing misfortunes of others—from the slapstick pratfalls of Jim Carrey and Amy Poehler to the self-inflicted humiliations of Martin Lawrence and Larry David—make us laugh even while they make us squirm?

I'll tell you why: because we've all been there. Shame is our common bond. It's our secret handshake. Shame isn't *one* of the things we all have in common; shame is the *main* thing we all have in common. It's the thing that reminds us that we're human, all too human. We've all gotten Cs on tests we told our friends we'd ace. We've all gone to school with stains on our shirts or bad haircuts, inadvertently belched in a hushed classroom, or raised our hands in class, only to forget the question we were trying to ask or answer. We've all said stupid, embarrassing, and hurtful things to people who meant us no harm, and we've all had unwholesome, selfish, or politically incorrect thoughts when piety was called for. We've all felt shame's scarlet sting on our cheeks.

The reason we laugh at the embarrassment of others is because we've been there too, and we're just glad that—this time—we're not the ones in the spotlight. When we laugh at the shame of others we're really laughing at ourselves. We're laughing out of relief, but we're also laughing out of solidarity.

So, if you're feeling ashamed about something you think no other respectable college student has ever experienced, think again. Sure, it all seems so very serious right now. But try, if you can, to find a little levity in your predicament. You'll discover that humor is more than the way shame relieves itself. You'll find that humor is shame's antidote.

And remember: you're not alone.

AM I SPECIAL?

Everyone wants to be special. Unfortunately, college is the place where the desire to feel special inevitably collides with reality. It turns out that your classmates are special too and that your professors are generally less smitten with you than your high school teachers and parents might have been. To add injury to insult, not everyone you want to bed or befriend will find you irresistible.

Some students find this collision of expectation with reality traumatic. They become overly disappointed with themselves. Worse, they worry that they've let down their parents.

The preferred way to overcome disappointment with yourself is by doing your best academically. Succeeding in school will help restore your self-esteem and make it easier for you to figure out where you're special and where you're not. Don't give up just because you feel overwhelmed, have to struggle, or get poor grades. Many of your classmates will be struggling too.

The worst way to reestablish your sense of specialness is to disdain the hard work of succeeding academically and to find some perverse way of distinguishing yourself, like becoming the campus player or coke dealer.

Dealing with your parents' real or perceived disappointment is more complicated. First, try to be open with your parents about your struggles. Give them the chance to deal with your anxieties as well as their own. All parents want their children to be successful and happy. But most will rise to the occasion when their children are floundering. Their regard for you will be increased, not decreased, by your candor, and they'll do their best to give you the support and reassurance you need. You'll feel relieved that they're not disillusioned with you, and they'll be glad you kept them in the loop.

If your parents are not able to work through their disappointment with you, it may be because they've never dealt with disappointments they have with themselves or with one of your siblings. They may have been unconsciously hoping that you would be the "good" child— the one who never had problems or who redeemed the family's honor—and you may have unconsciously sensed this. But that is their problem, not yours. You are under no obligation—and probably can't—make up for their unhappiness with their own lives or their disappointment with your sibling.

Figuring out how to feel special when that feeling collides with reality is one of the ways you learn to become an adult. Becoming independent of your parents is another. Although it's certainly easier to cope with blows to your specialness *with* your parents' help, doing so *without* their help may actually hasten the process of growing up. Either way, you'll end up being your own person—with your own internal resources for feeling special. And you'll be an adult.

FINISHING COLLEGE IS THE BEGINNING OF ADULTHOOD

Sooner or later you are going to leave college. You may pick up a nice, crisp diploma from the president or some other dignitary four years after setting foot on campus; you may have your degree mailed to you a year or two late after you finally turn in your overdue papers and finish your incompletes; you may never get your degree or get it many years later from a different institution. Sooner or later, however, you will leave college.

You will most likely be twenty-two, twenty-three, or twenty-four years old. You will be headed for a job, travel, further schooling, or your parents' basement. You may have clear goals that you prepared for throughout college or have absolutely no clue about what to do with the rest of your life. Your parents might be willing to help you out financially for a while or not. No matter the circumstance, finishing college is the beginning of adulthood.

How are you feeling? Are you feeling centered, hopeful, and confident or confused, anxious, and riddled with doubt? Whatever. It doesn't matter. You will find your way. Things have a way of working out. The wheel turns: those who were up are down and those who were down are up. Nobody escapes misfortune and no one has only bad luck.

Since ambivalence about leaving college and entering the adult world is normal, what you *don't* want to do is drive those feelings underground where they're no longer susceptible to reflection, reason, and reassurance. Feelings that are driven out of consciousness because of shame are often transformed when they finally resurface into symptoms whose origins are obscure and whose effects are consequently harder to deal with.

Here's how the unconscious fear of leaving college may come back to haunt you: instead of feeling anxious about life *post*graduation, you suddenly develop problems that require you to *postpone* graduation. For example, after managing to pull through your freshman and sophomore year by last-minute cramming, you discover during the second semester of your junior year that you've lost the will to work and have to drop two classes. Or, having been kept in check by antidepressants throughout college, your depression inexplicably flares up again in your senior year and becomes disabling.

In other words, the way your ambivalence about leaving college will announce itself is through the late development of a sudden and inexplicable problem that keeps you from graduating—except it *isn't* inexplicable because the timing of your problems is a dead giveaway.

Here's the sequence of your unconscious thoughts: It's my senior (or junior) year; I'm approaching the end of college; I'm *anxious* about entering the adult world; because I'm "supposed" to be more confident by this point in my life, I'm *ashamed* of my fear of entering the adult world; rather than *admit* I'm afraid of taking the next step (shameful), let me *avoid* taking the next step by developing a problem that will prevent me from graduating (less shameful because ostensibly "beyond my control"). So, low and behold, a problem "crops up" that postpones graduation.

Thus does shame convert distress into disability.

There's another telltale sign that you're dealing with ambivalence about growing up: your parents are suddenly back in your life again—

looking after you and worrying about you the way they did when you were a kid. They're picking you up and wiping away your tears like they did when you fell off your tricycle; they're shifting the focus of their attention from themselves back onto you like they did when you had trouble in middle school; they're taking it upon themselves to deal with the authorities (the doctors, the counselors, the deans) with whom, up till then, you'd been dealing on your own; most annoyingly, they're giving you gratuitous advice on how to live that you already know and resent being forced to listen to just because you're down.

Getting your parents involved again addresses one-half of the ambivalence about growing up by reassuring you that the safety net is still intact. But it aggravates the other side of the ambivalence—your desire to become independent—by making you feel incompetent when you're really not.

So don't be ashamed of your fear of leaving college and don't let it rob you of your confidence. Talk about your ambivalence with your parents if you need to. Talk about it with your friends who are going through the same thing if you want to. Talk about it with your therapist or your friendly thesis adviser if you have one. But have faith in your ability to cope with the transition to adulthood. Leaving college is only the first step anyway. And most of us who've tripped over the threshold have landed on our feet in the fullness of time.

ADVICE

You will hear plenty of advice when you finish college. Some of it will come from the commencement speaker at graduation, some will come from your parents and friends. Most of it will be good advice: Follow your dreams. Be responsible stewards of the planet. Leave the world a better place. Don't make money the principal reason for choosing your career. Spread human fellowship and love. Get a good haircut and good suit for job interviews. Think twice before marrying your first girlfriend or boyfriend. Be careful what you post on Facebook. Plastic!

Let me throw in my two bits.

First, be wary of seemingly innocuous comments made by acquaintances, friends, putative authorities, and self-styled experts that sound friendly and authoritative but have the effect of making you feel crummy.

Here are some examples of damaging remarks made to patients of mine—remarks that got buried in their memories but continued to affect them for many years:

An esteemed professor told a young woman who was having trouble in his organic chemistry course that she wasn't cut out to be a scientist. The young woman was crestfallen and considered switching her major to comp lit. But doing neuroscience research had been her lifelong dream. She retook organic chemistry over the subsequent summer, passed it, earned a PhD, and went on to work for a biotech company.

Another patient didn't fare so well. She too was struggling with organic chemistry and was told by her premed adviser that she wouldn't be able to succeed in medical school. Rather than persist, she abandoned her dream of becoming a doctor and switched to public health—not a bad field, but not what she had really wanted to do.

There are lots of examples of young people who have been discouraged from following challenging career paths because of some alleged defect in their personalities or aptitudes. What is regrettable is that most of the time these supposedly intractable defects can be overcome by hard work or further maturation. I've had patients discouraged from becoming investment bankers because they were told they weren't aggressive enough, from becoming psychologists because they weren't selfless enough, from becoming actors because they weren't talented enough, and from becoming lawyers because they weren't diligent enough. They all chose different careers and lived for many years with regret.

Sure, you could say that these young people should have ignored those negative comments and pursued their goals like the woman in the first example, who retook organic chemistry over the summer and became a neuroscientist. You could say that those who dropped out must have lacked the requisite fortitude to complete the arduous training programs these careers entail. You could even say that, if they were really cut out to do these jobs, they would have found a way to do them. And you would be right. Except that when you're young and uncertain and the people giving the advice seem to know about those careers, it's hard to ignore bad advice. It's even hard to recognize that the advice is bad! And, when the people giving the advice—parents, teachers, coaches, and friends—claim to know *you* (perhaps better even than you know yourself), who are you to disagree with them?

Watch out especially for comments that are made off the cuff, as an aside, or about someone else *like* you—they're the most insidiously harmful. Because they're harder to recognize and challenge, indirect and oblique comments have a way of embedding themselves in your psyche like a sliver that festers and can't be dislodged. You're pricked without even knowing it.

Here are some classics of the genre: a friend's mother boasts that her son is becoming an architect while you're "only" becoming a graphic designer—so, for the first time since the two of you have been friends, you begin to feel resentful of him and vaguely inferior. You're at a party and you notice someone roll her eyes at another girl's uninhibited dancing—so you stop dancing with joy to avoid the other girl's fate. When you're seven, your mother says you look fat in jeans and masculine with short hair—so you wear skirts and keep your hair long even as an adult. A friend remarks, ostensibly to be intimate, "You and I are different from the popular crowd; we're more serious"—so you reject overtures from the popular kids you might otherwise enjoy and join the Nietzsche club. An acquaintance sneers that people who use big words are conceited—so you dumb yourself down, that vegans are flaky—so you conceal your dietary quirks, that business people are only interested in money—so you become a social worker, or that strong-minded people don't really need to take psychiatric medication—so you stop taking your antidepressants and start to get panic attacks.

The absolute worst kinds of comments are those that stick a pin in your ego just when it's most inflated: you're singing with all your heart at the Christmas concert and the person beside you hisses that you're off-key, you've lost yourself in the part you're acting in the school play and someone in the wings whispers you're a ham, you're running a relay race and one of the boys on the sidelines observes that the fat on your thighs is quivering, or you're depicting the growth of a flower at your high school's modern dance performance and your brother starts laughing. These moments—the moments when you're feeling most alive and fulfilled, when you're expressing the best part of yourself without inhibition, when you're feeling special and trust that others are happy for you—these are the moments not only of greatest pleasure but also of greatest vulnerability. A pointed remark during one of those "up" moments (and what is it about such moments that attracts such cruelty?) can be devastating.

It's important to examine negative comments like these critically because they can alter the course of your life without your even being aware of it. You have to recognize them for what they are—received notions, conventional thinking, unexamined prejudices, passing shots, and pseudo-insightful put-downs—and understand the motives of the person making them—ignorance, envy, jealousy, competitiveness, the desire to fit in, and our old friend shame. Realizing the true nature of these banalities and the people who are making them is hard to do. The pronouncements themselves sound plausible and insightful, and the people making them often purport to be helpful and friendly. Since both the comments and the people making them have the ring of truth, they're hard to dismiss.

The best clue that you're being adversely affected by these covertly negative comments is that they make you feel crummy. They make you feel deflated, diminished, and disarmed. You feel more envious and competitive than you did beforehand, yet ashamed of feeling that way because the comments that occasioned those feelings were made "innocently" or about someone else or were meant to be "helpful." Above all, you feel that your opportunities have gotten fewer and your horizons more distant. Your light has been dimmed.

In short, passing comments are hard to detect and they're hard to dismiss. They're subtle and insidious. They're often made by people who are influential, authoritative, and even well intentioned—close friends, admired peers, teachers, advisers, job supervisers, parents, and therapists. They have the ring of truth. They leave you feeling dazed and confused. They have more influence than they deserve. They're limiting rather than freeing.

Because digs like these are subtle and hard to dismiss, you have to confront them using a ton of reason and a pound of rage. Are the comments true or do they merely *sound* true? Are they based on real understanding and insight or only on conventional wisdom and prejudice? Does the person making the comments really know what he's talking about or is he talking through his hat? Has she given the matter actual thought or is she just shooting from the hip? Even if true in general, are the comments applicable to *you*—and are they applicable to you *at this stage of your life*? Do the comments expand your options or shrink them?

It may or may not be helpful to question the motives of the person making the comments. Because the purity of a person's motives is not so easy to determine, because mistaken judgments about people's motives can lead to paranoia and unnecessary conflict, and because pure motives don't guarantee valid insights anyway, you're still required to evaluate the comments on their merits. And in that task you have to use your own reasoned judgment.

Your Mother's Advice Was Not Always Wrong

Most people love their mothers. But there is one thing mothers do that is just infuriating: they give you good advice that's a pain in the neck to follow.

They tell you to eat a good breakfast (and lunch and dinner), to consume vegetables and avoid junk food. They tell you to get a good night's sleep—to go to bed and wake up early. They tell you to do first things first—to do your homework before going out to have fun. They tell you to exercise regularly, to see the doctor when you're not feeling well, to avoid drugs, and to drink moderately. They tell you to practice safe sex, to avoid abusive relationships, and to ask for help when you're having trouble.

Infuriating!

Because you know these recommendations are good for you—and often tough to follow in college—it's really irritating when your mother reminds you of them. It's irritating even when she *doesn't* remind you of them because you know what she's thinking anyway and because you're already irritated with yourself.

The funny thing is that when therapists give the same advice (they call it self-care) it seems much wiser and less infuriating.

AM I IN THE RIGHT THERAPY?

Since the most authoritative person you're likely to receive advice from is your therapist, it's worth exploring the question *Am I in the right therapy?* Which translates to *Is the treatment I'm getting the right one for my problem? And, more important, is the therapist I'm seeing the right one for me?*

Let's look at how you got here.

Most college students entering therapy for the first time will contact the student health service or a practitioner in the community and make an appointment. Sometimes you'll have the name of a specific person to see, often you won't. Either way you'll have some trepidation while sitting in the waiting room: Will I like this person? Will she be able to help me? Will I trust him enough to be able to open up?

The door opens and your therapist invites you into her office. Naturally, you have first impressions: she seems young or old, chilly or warm, approachable or intimidating, attractive or unattractive, professional or unprofessional, etc. You know you have to reserve judgment on the relevance of all these issues because first impressions can be wrong and the most unlikely therapist can turn out to be the most helpful and because you're bringing your own prejudices to the situation and those prejudices themselves may be part of the therapy.

So you're trying to keep an open mind, but, of course, your impressions are your impressions—and, as I've said before about trusting yourself, in the final analysis you're going to have to rely on them.

But you're not there yet; it's still the first meeting and much has yet to be decided.

The first thing the therapist should do is to find out why you've come. And here is where the responsibility shifts to you and, in a sense, stays with you. It's your job to describe your predicament—your symptoms, your feelings, your thoughts, your behaviors, your history, your reactions and interactions with other people (including to the therapist when relevant)—as clearly and openly as you can. The therapist should help you to do this by guiding you and asking questions when necessary, but she shouldn't have to do your work for you by pulling teeth.

When the therapist has completed his evaluation (which may take more than one appointment), he should be able to tell you what he thinks is going on with you and how best to deal with it. He may describe your problem in psychiatric terms ("I think you're suffering from an anxiety disorder"), in psychological terms ("You seem to be disappointed that you're not working as hard on your schoolwork as you know you can"), or in social terms ("You're struggling to find friends you feel comfortable with"). But, however he describes your problem, it should resonate with you. If it doesn't, you should tell him in what way your impression differs from his and see if the two of you can get on the same wavelength.

The next thing the therapist should do is to make a recommendation about treatment. This may involve psychotherapy, medication, or a combination of the two. It may occasionally involve just reassurance and no therapy. If the therapist can't provide the type of therapy you need, or can only provide part of it, she may refer you to someone else. The therapist should describe what the therapy entails, length, frequency, and cost of appointments, and her cancellation policy. You should work out *together* what the goals of therapy will be and try to reach an understanding of what each of you will endeavor to do in order to achieve those goals. If you have questions or reservations, express them. Don't reject a reasonable treatment plan out of hand, but don't accept it just because she's the expert and you're "the one with the problem." The arrangements have to work for both of you.

In most cases, you'll get to end of the evaluation feeling *reasonably* confident that the practitioner you've met with will be able to help you. You'll make a follow-up appointment. And the treatment will begin.

But what if you still have reservations about the therapist or the therapy after the initial visit? What then? Well, first of all, some reservations are appropriate: you're putting your well-being in this stranger's hands and you don't necessarily have an objective way to determine whether he's on the right track or is the right person. Discuss your concerns with the therapist and see how he deals with them. Are his responses helpful and reassuring? Do you learn something useful about yourself from the discussion? Do you feel more and more comfortable and in sync with the therapist as the treatment progresses? Is it getting easier to be open in the treatment? Do you feel increasingly understood?

Even in the very best therapies, things occasionally go off track. The therapist makes a gaffe, misses an appointment, forgets some pertinent detail of your history, seems out of sorts, or says something irritating. Naturally, this is very disconcerting. It makes you wonder if she really understands you. But these disconcerting moments, properly handled, can also be rare opportunities. They can lead to unexpected breakthroughs—breakthroughs that could not have occurred any other way and that deepen your self-understanding and your connection to the therapist. At the very least, since slipups and failures of empathy are inevitable in human relations, the therapist's gaffes provide you with a controlled environment in which to learn how to deal with them.

Of course, every modality of therapy has its own unique therapist-patient or therapist-client interaction. And even within a particular modality, every therapist operates a little bit differently. In behavioral therapies, like cognitive-behavioral therapy (CBT) and dialect-behavioral therapy (DBT), the therapist acts more like a teacher or guide, pointing out dysfunctional patterns of thinking and behavior and suggesting alternative coping mechanisms. She may assign homework or other exercises to help you build new ways of dealing with feelings and relationships. Therapists in behavioral therapies focus more on teaching skills and less on providing insight or exploring underlying motivation.

Behavior-oriented therapists tend to be pretty supportive and directive. But support and education are part of *all* therapies to some degree. Insight-oriented therapists too strive to create a safe, nonjudgmental environment in which clients can explore their thoughts and feelings. Practitioners who do psychoanalytic, interpersonal, and problem-focused therapies also try to point out dysfunctional patterns of behavior. But, instead of trying to teach new ways of responding or new coping skills as behavioral therapists do, exploratory therapists try to discover the earlier context in which these dysfunctional patterns arose and *were* "functional." The assumption is that, armed with these insights, you will be able to achieve a more truthful understanding of yourself and of other people. And that, unencumbered by the past, you'll be free to try different, healthier ways of living.

Although behavior therapies have been validated in outcome studies more extensively than exploratory therapies, both types of therapy have been shown to be helpful for most of the common problems with which students present. Good therapists often employ elements of the other modality when they're treating patients—behaviorists sometimes offer insight and psychoanalysts sometimes offer advice.

The choice of therapy should be worked out in concert with the person evaluating you. In some cases, the therapy will be matched to the nature of the problem. But, in many cases, the therapy will be matched to the aptitudes and preferences of the therapist or client. Provided that the therapy is effective for the problem, that the therapist is adept at the therapy, and that the patient is comfortable with both therapist and therapy, either approach to choosing the treatment can work.

So, after you've been properly evaluated and begun therapy in good faith, how do you answer the question am I in the right therapy?

The short answer is: if you still have to ask the question, you're probably not.

The long answer involves being able to answer in the affirmative a series of further questions:

- Do you feel comfortable with the therapist, and she with you? Are you able to satisfactorily work out differences and disagreements? You should respect your therapist but not be intimidated by her.
- Do you feel understood? Does the therapist "get" you and appreciate you? Even though much of your joint attention in therapy must necessarily focus on your weaknesses, does your therapist seem to recognize your strengths?
- Are you gradually starting to feel better? Are you making headway toward achieving the goals you established at the outset or during the course of therapy? You shouldn't expect to leave every session feeling better, but is the trend line positive?
- Most important, is your life getting better? Are you functioning more effectively academically and interpersonally? Are you feeling happier and more adult?

If you've been able to answer yes to most of those questions, you may want to persevere with the treatment. But if you haven't been able to answer yes to those questions, or you've discussed your concerns with your therapist and still don't feel comfortable with what's happening in the treatment, you should ask for a second opinion or tell the therapist you plan to stop seeing him. Every practitioner of every stripe and level of experience has clients who drop out or move on. It's OK. It's OK for the therapist. And it's OK for you. You have to do what's best for you—and you have to trust your own judgment about what that is. It's your therapy and your life.

You Can Handle the Truth

The foundation of any good therapy—and of any good life—is discovering and acknowledging the truth about the world, about your parents and friends, and, most important, about yourself.

I could almost say that it's not possible to have a full life *without* discovering and acknowledging the truth. Yes there are beliefs and fantasies that make life more livable. I might feel better believing there's an afterlife or that what goes around comes around. I might like the fantasy that this book will help a lot of people or that I'll sell enough copies to afford a house on the beach. But having those beliefs or fantasies doesn't detract from my ability to discern, in my daily life, what's real and what's not, what's true and what's an illusion.

And, yes, we sometimes need little white lies and petty vanities to get through the day. But those little white lies don't detract from our ability to live in reality. Like courtesy, tact, and charm, they increase the world's store of harmony and grace and reduce the abrasiveness of human contact. By the time we're in college, we ought to be able to tell the difference between the small hypocrisies that make life livable and the substantive lies that spread confusion and suffering—and we should be trying our best to act on that knowledge.

So let me make a point about the truth—it's *not* brutal. It's not brutal because the important truths, those that pertain to us and to the people in our lives, are usually complicated and nuanced. That's why brutal honesty, whether directed toward yourself or toward others, is usually a species of lie. At best it's a partial truth that pretends to see only the harsh part of the reality and not the softening part that gives the truth balance and makes it whole. As I said, the truth is usually complicated and nuanced. To claim otherwise is to impose an agenda on the truth—to use "truth telling" as a form of propaganda or punishment. (I keep saying "usually" because sometimes—as in child molestation or abuse, untreated parental alcoholism, or domestic violence—the truth is brutal and has to be faced up to without prevarication or mitigation.)

Let's take a trivial but common example of how a partial truth can be used brutally. Suppose you wake up one morning after eating a whole pizza the night before, look at yourself in the mirror, and say *You're a disgusting pig!*

Are you telling yourself the whole truth? No, you're not. You might not even be telling a partial truth. What you're doing is being unkind to yourself to give the *appearance* of telling the truth—probably to evade a more difficult and important truth. By calling yourself "disgusting" instead of "occasionally self-indulgent," you're pulling a fast one. You could be trying to atone for your carbohydrate overdose the night before, giving yourself permission to indulge in another pizza that morning, excusing your crankiness to your roommate, or hoping to elicit reassurance from your mother when you call her to complain. But, whatever your agenda, what you're *not* doing is telling the whole truth—which means that you're not really telling the truth at all.

Now, obviously, if you persisted in telling yourself these brutal untruths, you could make yourself quite depressed. Then your depression too would be a based on a lie. And you'd only be able to get better when you began telling yourself the actual truth—which is that sometimes you overindulge in fattening foods and that if you persist in doing so you will be unhappy with the consequences. Telling yourself the truth in this case would help you to take responsibility for yourself and to gain more control of your life. Telling yourself the truth would help you to become an adult.

Let's take a more important example. Suppose it's your ambition to become a lawyer, but you're intimidated about the amount of work required to get the grades to get into law school. If you were truthful about your fear of doing the work, you might feel motivated to try a little harder to do a good job on your assignments. But if you were unwilling to face up to the truth, you might tell yourself that you didn't really want to be a lawyer after all, that it was something you were doing just to please your father, who's a lawyer. You could probably find something else to do that makes you happy, but, by rationalizing your unwillingness to work and lying to yourself about your motivation, you would have walked away from your probably genuine ambition to be a lawyer.

Just as a general observation, when you say *I'm only doing this because my parents want me to*, a sure tip-off that you're being dishonest with yourself is that the "this" you're unhappy about doing is unpleasant or difficult. If you seem to have no trouble overcoming parental expectations when the activity in question is pleasant and easy (like smoking pot or spending an afternoon playing video games), then you shouldn't make the excuse that you're having trouble overcoming parental expectations when the activity is unpleasant and difficult (like handing in assignments on time or trying to get good grades).

Because you almost always know when you're lying to yourself, *discovering* the truth is less difficult than *acknowledging* the truth. All it really takes to discover the truth is listening to your inner voice. Your inner voice is usually pretty clear and reasonable. It will tell you, for example, that you're *not* disgusting, merely self-indulgent, or that it's really *your* ambition to be a lawyer, not your father's. You almost always know when you're lying to yourself.

Acknowledging the truth is harder because it entails action. Once you acknowledge the truth, you know you have to act on it, otherwise you'll feel disappointed in yourself and unhappy. Acknowledging the truth means, if you want to be healthy, that you have stop indulging in so much pizza eating and, if you want to get into law school, that you have to work harder. Acknowledging the truth means you have to change. And change is hard.

But acknowledging the truth also means accepting the things you *can't* change. It means recognizing your shortcomings and trying to find a reasonable balance between accepting and improving them. And it means accepting the reasonable shortcomings of others. Acknowledging the truth means being kinder to yourself and to others while holding yourself and them to reasonable standards.

People who are able to discover and acknowledge the truth are happier with themselves and more at home in the world. They live in reality and deal with the world realistically. The discipline of discovering and acknowledging the truth is not something you will fully achieve in college—it's a lifelong challenge. But college is not too early a time to start. Because, by the time you're in college, you can handle the truth.

BE BRAVE

Which leads me to my final piece of advice: be brave. It takes bravery to discover and acknowledge the truth. And it takes bravery to learn to trust your own judgment, especially when it conflicts with received wisdom or the prevailing dogma.

How do you learn to trust your own judgment? By assuming—despite your own desire to fit in with the thinking of everyone else—that your *honest* perceptions, impressions, ideas, and conclusions have merit. And by assuming that your doubts, insecurities, errors, and embarrassing gaffes—even your gigantic blunders—are normal.

It's hard to feel normal when your feelings or perceptions appear to conflict with those of the people around you. And they may *not* be normal. They may be psychopathic or delusional. They may be dangerous or mistaken. But they may also be truer and more perceptive than what you're *supposed* to believe. I'm not saying you should *act* on every judgment, particularly if it will result in suffering for you or for others. But you shouldn't be afraid to examine how you feel *as if* it were normal just because others might frown upon it.

Be skeptical of your own opinions and consider the other side—certainly. Play devil's advocate with yourself—sure. Bounce your thoughts off other people—by all means. But, when push comes to shove, be brave—trust your own judgment.

Unsure about whether to support an unpopular cause or political candidate, ask your boss for a raise, confront a friend or coworker who's been giving you a hard time, wear white after Labor Day? Be brave—trust your own judgment.

More important, if your view of your childhood differs from that of your parents or therapist—be brave: trust your own judgment. If your understanding of how the world works differs from that of your professors or your closest friends—be brave: trust your own judgment. If you don't love your boyfriend enough to marry him—even though he's "perfect for you," everyone says you're a fool for hesitating and tells you that you have a problem committing—be brave: trust your own judgment.

You may turn out to be wrong. You may have regrets. Your feelings and ideas may eventually evolve in the direction of the conventional view. You may realize you were more of a pain in the butt as a child than you cared to remember when you were initially trying to form your judgment of your childhood. You may come to agree with your professors or your friends about how the world works. You may realize after he's happily married with two kids that you should have grabbed your boyfriend while he was available. But, in the meantime, you have no choice but to trust your own judgment.

Of course, you must follow the mandate to discover and acknowledge the truth. You shouldn't kid yourself about important things or lie to yourself merely to assert your independence. Your life is too important to make yourself the creature of other people's expectations by rewarding or dashing *their* hopes instead of following your *own*. But, once you've searched your soul and tried to be as honest with yourself as you can, you have to be brave and trust your own judgment.

You can—and sometimes should—consult your parents, your trusted adviser, your spiritual pastor, or your best friend to give yourself a reality check, but when it comes to deciding what you really believe and what you really want to do, you have to learn to trust your own judgment above that of all others.

It's hard to trust your own judgment. You're young. You're relatively inexperienced. You have a mortal fear of making a fool of yourself. You're sure you missed the class where the manual on how to live was given out, because everyone else but you seems to know the right thing to do. And, despite having been warned, you've made mistakes, some of which have been doozies.

But you have no choice. You *have* to be brave and you *have* to trust your own judgment because you're no longer a kid. You're at the beginning of becoming an adult.

And now I'm going to let you in on a big secret: being an adult is *way* better than being a college student.

For Parents

Do Parents Have a Role?

As a psychiatrist and parent, I categorically reject the idea that, when your child turns eighteen, you, the parents, have completed your job (presumably badly!) and been rendered obsolete. I reject the idea that, despite their legal majority and rights, most eighteen or twenty-two year olds are fully fledged and ready to fly completely on their own. I reject the idea that your college-aged children no longer have anything to gain from your wisdom and experience. I especially reject the idea that the small army of experts you'll have to contend with when your kid has a problem (including not just therapists and college administrators but also journalists and political commentators) necessarily knows better than you how to help your son or daughter.

Ideas about child rearing and the role of parents in preventing or producing psychological problems change over time—and not always for sound scientific reasons. Often as not, these trends are based on political fads. Should the mother take time off from work to raise her children or is she better off developing a career that serves as a model for them? Which situation—divorce or a high level of marital conflict—is more harmful? What's the best way to instill a work ethic in a child—strict discipline or giving her freedom to follow her passion? No one knows for sure, but the debate generates a lot of heat.

One idea that never seems to go out of fashion, despite common sense and a growing body of evidence to the contrary, is the idea that the problems of the child can be laid at the doorstep of the parents. So, if you happen to have a kid who is troubled, smokes too much pot, or is an underachiever, therapists on one side of the debate or the other will be tempted to blame you.

Before I'm roundly dismissed as a quack and an idiot, let me say that, of course, parents and their child-rearing practices have an effect on their children. Some parents *do* abuse or mistreat or misunderstand and warp their children. Some parents *are* negligent or selfish or dense. Some parents *are* unfit to be parents and should never have had children. But, in my experience, these parents are few and far between. This is especially true of the parents whose children manage to make it into college.

All parents make mistakes and do harm to their children. Even the most loving and supportive parents can say and do awful things out of ignorance or anger. I'm not trying to excuse or condone the things parents do, even inadvertently, that end up harming their children. I make my living examining those events, understanding their consequences, and trying to put them into perspective. I'm well aware that some things parents do may be unforgivable. And I offer no whitewash for those pernicious words and deeds. But, as a good parent (and as a fair-minded kid), one thing you have to keep in mind is that not everything your child does—and this applies to her achievements as well as her failures—is your responsibility. You wouldn't take all the credit and you shouldn't take all the blame.

Before College Begins

The Gap Year

More and more students are taking a year off between high school and college to travel, perform community or military service, or work.

This is almost always a good thing. The student gets a chance to take a break from academic work and recharge his batteries while, at the same time, becoming more independent and mature. Most schools allow accepted students to defer matriculation for one year. Some students take the opportunity to upgrade their credentials and reapply to schools that have rejected them. After a year or more in the "real world," most students return to their studies more motivated and focused than they would otherwise have been, and more determined to get as much out of their college experience as they can.

Many students also take a year off *during* university. A leave of absence allows them time to figure out why they're in college and to grow up a bit more before continuing their education. Most schools permit a year off without penalty. Time off from college is so common that even *U.S. News and World Report* uses six years, not four, as their yardstick for ranking a college's graduation rate.

The Lazy Student

You might want to refer to chapter 2, "Academic Problems," for a fuller discussion of laziness. Suffice it to say here that laziness is a complex problem. It's a fact of human psychology that affects all of us to one degree or another, and it's a trait that varies normally across the population. Most lazy students have been lazy all the way through school. If they're bright and charming, they may have been able to get good marks, especially earlier in their education, without having had to overcome their laziness. However, when they hit high school, and definitely when they hit college, the workload increases to the point where they can no longer fake it. Their laziness gets reflected in their marks, and, unless they learn to overcome it, their laziness becomes an impediment to their success.

There are some things you can do to reduce your child's temptation to give in to his laziness. Exposing him to cultural resources and extracurricular activities, encouraging reading and discussion, turning off the TV, treating learning disabilities and emotional problems when they arise, limiting alcohol use in the home, building self-esteem through achievement and support, instilling discipline both by encouragement and example, and recognizing his individuality rather than imposing your dreams on him—all of these interventions will help to remove impediments to your child's fulfillment and success. You have to be flexible, resourceful, thick-skinned, and patient. The results may not be immediately apparent. They might not even be apparent until your child has become an adult himself. But doing the right things *might* help. And *not* doing the right things might prevent a remediable problem from being remedied.

AFTER COLLEGE BEGINS

Normal Stuff: Separation and Growing-up

As every student and parent knows, college is about more than just getting a degree; it's about learning how to become an adult. I don't think that most students will have completed that transition by the time they graduate with a bachelor's degree, but they will have made significant progress. They will be more independent and self-sufficient and their worldviews will be more autonomous. Sometimes their progress toward adulthood will put them at odds with you; sometimes it will put them more in harmony with you. Either way, their interactions with you while they're undergoing this transition will require sensitivity and open-mindedness on both sides—but especially on your part because, after all, you already *are* adult.

In dealing with the vicissitudes of your child's transition to adulthood, you won't handle everything correctly—and neither will she. Your child is under no obligation to make everything easy for you (though it would be nice if she didn't make everything difficult), and you can be pretty sure that she won't. One moment she'll be incredibly mature, self-reliant, and confident; the next moment she'll be a basket case. Regression is normal—as long as it's followed by progression. One moment he'll be loving and sweet; the next moment he'll be a monster. Hostility helps him free himself from dependence on you—as long as it's tempered and temporary. Sometimes she'll want your help, sometimes she won't. Knowing how to respond to the ups and downs of your child's moods and the two-steps-forward-one-step-back of her march to adulthood requires you to keep a cool head and an eye on the big picture.

The transition to adulthood is neither uniform nor smooth. If your son wants to come home every weekend for the first semester he's in college, let him. Don't belittle him or chastise him. He'll stay at school when he's ready. Yes, his coming home may prolong the time it takes him to feel at home there—and you can gently point that out to him. But he'll find it easier to stay at school if he knows he can to it at his own pace.

If your daughter wants to take her stuffed animals to the dorm, gains ten pounds the first semester, calls you every night and falls apart before every menstrual period, let her. There's no need to over-react. She's probably behaving more maturely with her peers than with you and she'll likely regain her usual poise as soon as she's made a few friends.

College is a place where young people can reinvent themselves. They can shed the parts of their identities they've outgrown or dis-like and experiment with new identities that more truly express who they feel they are or who they would like to be. Because fewer people know what they were like in the past, they're freer to try on different ways of thinking and behaving at college than they were at home. They're less straitjacketed by having to live up to their old reputa-tions or please old onlookers. This is a rare and wonderful thing. The worst thing we can do as parents is to force them back into that old straitjacket by responding to them as if they were still the same im-mature kid they were when they left.

If you can remember what you were like at their age, you'll know that college students behave one way when they're with you and an-other way when they're with their peers. You daughter can hang up after a tearful phone call with you that leaves you ready to call 911, then be perfectly calm and happy when she goes out with her friends. She can mope around watching TV and eating junk when she's at home on a break, then get down to work and exercise daily when she's back at school. (Even we middle-aged adults regress a little when we visit our parents, so why would we expect our twenty-somethings not to do so?) Sometimes you can't help it though: you just have to tell her to get off the couch and go outside or you'll go nuts. But, most of the time, confronting her regressive behavior is useless: it humiliates her and produces unnecessary conflict in the household with very little to show for it.

The hardest thing for parents to figure out is when to back off. If you're attentive to the clues—nonverbal as well as verbal—your child is giving you, however, he'll *tell* you whether or not he wants you to get involved. There will come a time when you'll have to let your child flounder and cope. Doing so will require great fortitude and trust on your part and great bravery and resourcefulness on his.

Lance had stopped working hard academically in his junior year after getting back a disappointing result on his LSAT test. Never the most diligent student, Lance had still managed to maintain a GPA around 3.5 with middling effort. Lance had nurtured an ambition to be a lawyer, like his successful father, ever since his parents had told him that his precocious argumentativeness would suit him for the profession. He *had* studied hard for the LSAT, hoping to get into a top-ten law school, but his mark of 165 made that goal seem unrealistic.

Unwilling to apply to any but "the top" law schools, Lance saw no reason to keep his grades up. He dropped a course for lack of attendance and became increasingly depressed. He slept all day, smoked pot all night, and bathed infrequently. He made remarks about not seeing a future—remarks that made his parents worry he might be suicidal. After much discussion between them, his parents decided to pick Lance up from school one Friday and bring him home—maybe for the weekend, maybe for the term.

Once home, Lance and his parents spoke on and off for the next two days. They told him that even with his current LSAT score (which was quite respectable, they reminded him) he'd be able to get into a very fine law school—if that was what *he* decided to do. They reassured him that it didn't matter to *them* whether or not he became a lawyer if another career interested him more. They told him there was no rush for him to figure out what to do after he graduated. They said that it would be all right with them if he needed to take time off from school to regroup. And, finally, they told him they'd support him no matter *what* he chose to do with his life.

On Sunday afternoon, Lance told his parents that he wanted to go back to school.

"My friends are all there," he told them. "And I can think more clearly when I'm in my own space."

Lance's parents were still worried about him. But they felt pretty certain he was not a suicide risk. "We respect your courage and your desire to deal with this on your own," they told him. "All we ask is that you please just keep us informed about how you're doing."

Lance agreed and returned to school that evening. He continued to struggle with his sudden ambivalence about law school, but he cleaned himself up, got down to work, and pulled up his grades.

By allowing him to cope with his crisis on his own, Lance's parents put their relationship with him on a more mature footing and gave him the chance to start a new phase in his voyage toward adulthood. Having pulled himself up by his bootstraps, Lance felt more ready to face life after graduation on his own. And, having had their faith in him rewarded, Lance's parents felt good about their careful and respectful intervention—and very proud of him.

Tough Stuff: The Student Who Is Floundering Academically

How can you help your son or daughter in college who is not living up to his potential? How do you deal with her unwillingness to do her schoolwork or to remedy her low grades? Should you try nagging, issue subtle reminders about work you know he has to get done, threaten to pull him out of school until he gets more motivated? Should you treat your college-age children as adults—let them struggle with their academic problems and deal with the consequences on their own, without trying to rescue them?

Each situation and each kid will require her own unique solution, of course, but there are some general principles that might be helpful:

First, floundering, struggling, even failure are not without their educational value—but only if the struggling student eventually recovers. As an adult trying to help your child deal with her academic travails, your first task is to do what you can to keep her from completely giving up. She may need to transfer, take time off, work for a while, take a medical leave of absence, take incompletes, or return to school later as a mature student, but you want to make sure she doesn't think that running aground academically in her early twenties means that her academic life cannot be salvaged. As I've said before, it is the genius of the American university system that it allows students multiple opportunities to complete their education. (And, it should be added, it is the genius of the American workplace that it hires graduates not only from elite colleges but also from a host of postsecondary institutions.)

Second, you will be angry and disappointed that your kid isn't performing, especially when you know she's capable of excelling but isn't doing the work needed to do so. You'll be tempted to scold, cajole, remind, nag, criticize, and check up on her to keep her going. But what will be the result? She *might* pull up her socks temporarily because of your nagging, but when she reverts to her old bad habits, as she inevitably will because she still hasn't taken ownership of her academic responsibilities, she won't tell you about it until she's past the point of no return. No one wants to be told what to do when they're afraid they won't be able to do it. And most people don't want to disappoint their parents, cause them pain, or waste their money. So nagging and its associated behaviors rarely work. In any case, since both you and your child want her to become an independent adult, continuing to act as her coach is ultimately counterproductive.

It might be more prudent to let her take time off from school before she's blighted her transcript; give her time to grow up a little and become more responsible by taking a job, expressing faith in her ability to recover from her academic difficulties so that she doesn't give up; then, when she's ready, support her return to school.

Last, *get tuition reimbursement insurance before each term!* This is private insurance that reimburses up to 90 percent of the tuition, room, board, and required fees not refunded by the college in the event that a student withdraws because of illness (including emotional illness), accident, or death. Tuition reimbursement insurance should *not* be confused with life insurance policies that guarantee to pay a student's tuition in the event of a *parent's* death. (It might make sense to get both kinds of policies, but it is essential to get tuition reimbursement insurance.) Most colleges will reimburse 90 percent of the tuition costs if a student withdraws within the first week. After that, the percentage decreases dramatically. Tuition reimbursement insurance pays the difference between what the college reimburses and what the total cost is for the term.

College financial services offices usually send out an application for tuition reimbursement insurance about one month before the school year begins. If you haven't received an application by then, call the college and get a referral to the company that provides this insurance right away. The application has to be completed and funded before the start of classes. Tuition reimbursement insurance costs between $100 and $200 per term. Considering the high cost of college and the unpredictability of life, it's a good investment.

An Aside to Faculty

Professors and academic advisers have a role to play here too. Instructors of wayward students should take the initiative to e-mail the student who is missing classes or not turning in assignments. You should let him know you want him to return to class, whether he feels fully prepared or not. Invite him to meet with you one on one. Make an effort to get to know him. If he's "gifted but lazy," he may be afraid to try and fail. Figure out how to help him channel his narcissism into productive and realistic pursuits rather than grandiose and self-destructive ones. Because many of you were "gifted and lazy" yourselves when you were undergraduates, you may be at risk of projecting your own self-reproach and hard-won self-discipline onto your students and of adopting a stance that is overly harsh—or overly permissive. Of course, you have to uphold standards and be impartial. In fact, it's dismaying to students, including students who are floundering, when rules are applied inequitably. But most students, *especially* those who want to be special, would like to be able to do their work and be successful. They're not looking for charity (generally); they're looking for a chance to redeem themselves. A nuanced blend of reasonable expectations, friendly encouragement, and concrete suggestions is more likely to be helpful than excessive punitiveness, leniency, or reproach. But *any* intervention is better than none at all.

Dealing With Your Own Feelings

The normal reaction when you find out your kid is floundering in college is a mixture of panic, fear, anger, guilt, and embarrassment. The panic and fear have to do with your child—concern for his welfare and future. (I'll deal with those feelings later.) The anger, guilt, and embarrassment have to do with you—the blow to *your* hopes and self-esteem—and have much less to do with your child. It is completely normal to want your child to succeed and make something of herself. It's normal to want to be seen as a good parent whose kids are thriving and happy. Neither of those feelings is evidence of "living through your children." It's *not* normal, however, to expect your child to go through her youth—especially through college —without some kind of problem. If your child has managed to make it through high school without a hitch, don't be dismayed if she runs into trouble in college—it happens to even the best and brightest students.

As you well know, every person has problems sooner or later. No one's path is straight onward and upward. Every child and every adult has ups and downs, successes and failures. If your child is floundering in school, it doesn't mean you've failed as a parent. It doesn't mean that it's your fault or that you're responsible. You don't have to hang your head in shame or start doubting yourself. You child is, to some (increasingly large) extent, responsible for her own predicament. Some things—mental illness, a crazy roommate, a poor fit with the college—may be outside her control. But many things—doing her schoolwork, looking after her health, exercising reasonable judgment—are within her control. You are *not* necessarily responsible for causing her problems. You *are* responsible for trying to help her solve them (but not by solving them yourself).

Let me begin with the same sort of advice I gave your wayward offspring: don't panic; don't despair; don't give up. But don't ignore a brewing problem either. The colleges, the legal system, and, of course, your kids will all tell you that college students are adults. Don't believe it. They are proto-adults. Certainly you want to encourage their developing independence and autonomy and respect their privacy. And certainly you sometimes have to let them make their own mistakes and fall on their faces. But don't be cowed by the admonition to let them screw up their lives because it's the only way they're going to learn to be adults. First, it isn't true that kids have to hit a brick wall in order to learn. Second, it isn't true that kids necessarily learn by suffering the consequences of their decisions: Very often they *don't* learn; they just suffer.

I don't mean to imply that some struggle and adversity in life isn't inevitable and even desirable: It can strengthen character and build legitimate confidence and self-reliance. But college provides enough formative adversity on its own. There is little to be gained by adding the trauma of failure and defeat—if it can be avoided. Permitting your child to blight his future for the sake of a lesson he could have learned in a less damaging way is unnecessary and gratuitously harsh. You have to try to help them—if they'll let you!

Dealing With Your Kid

And if they'll let you *know!* Part of the problem is that college students are often too ashamed to ask for help when they need it. And, because their expectations of their parents are contradictory, they're especially ashamed to ask for help from *you*. What are their contradictory feelings? Well, on one hand, they want you to view them as independent adults. On the other hand, they want you to figure out that they're hurting without having to actually verbalize it: they want to convey their misery by giving suggestive hints, taking poor care of themselves and pouting, like when they were little. Sometimes college students feel outraged when they're treated like kids and sometimes they feel outraged when they're not.

In theory, there ought to be a contract between you and your college-age kids that says the following: they agree to keep you informed of their progress on a regular basis and to seek help early when problems arise. You agree to create the conditions that will make it possible for them to do so by trying not to be intrusive or judgmental. In practice, things are much messier and more ad hoc.

Sometimes—often—you'll be confronted with a fait accompli that you hadn't expected or been warned about. By the time you're brought into the picture, your kid will already have dropped a class, gone on academic probation, withdrawn from school, been arrested by the campus police, taken an overdose, or consented to unprotected sex. You'll be angry and frightened. You'll want to shout at him. You'll want to take him by the shoulders and shake him. You'll want to ask him what he was thinking. You'll want to berate him for not coming to you sooner when the crisis could have been prevented or remedied.

Don't do it. You may not be able to hold back completely, but try to exercise restraint. It's tempting to say that *you* would have behaved more responsibly at your kid's age. Perhaps you would have. But you and your kid are different people living in a different time. Try to put yourself in your kid's shoes—not your *own* shoes as a college student, but your *kid's* shoes now.

Keep your focus on solving the problem. Trust your instincts and judgment. Be responsive. Be self-critical. Make sure you're being honest with yourself and your kid. But don't be cowed by him or by anyone else.

Expect some resistance. (Remember her guilt and shame.) Your kid is humiliated that she's let you down, wasted your money, and blemished her record. She's bound to feel defensive. Antagonism allows her to act as if you're to blame and (she hopes) keeps your criticism at bay. Beneath the antagonism, however, she knows she's responsible for her predicament and realizes that you're trying to help. Properly managed, crises like these can help make your relationship with her closer and more adult.

Dealing with Your Spouse's Feelings

If child-rearing disagreements are a large source of conflict between husbands and wives in good times, imagine how much heat they generate during bad times—like when their child is depressed, flunking out of college, or abusing drugs.

"You were too indulgent!" shouts the father. "You were too harsh!" counters the mother. When your kid is in crisis you want it all to go away—and you want someone to blame.

Try not to blame each other. First, as a matter of fact, it is rarely the case that one (or either) parent is to blame. (Unfortunately, the situation is further complicated when parents are divorced or have an adversarial marriage and, as a consequence, can't agree on how to raise their child or on how to come up with a coherent approach to dealing with his problems). Second, conflict between the two of you is threatening to your already worried child and, at the same time, gives him an opening to pit one of you against the other.

More important, try not to blame each other *in front of* your child. If you slip up and say something you shouldn't—feelings are running high after all—you should apologize publicly to your spouse and remind your child that, as parents, the two of you respect each other and are in fundamental agreement. Most family members, including the child in question, are able to put these intemperate outbursts in the correct perspective. If your child tries to exploit the apparent conflict between the two of you, however, nip it in the bud. It is far worse for your child to have the means to manipulate or drive a wedge between the two of you than for you to score a short-term victory over your spouse by contriving to be seen as the "good" parent.

Hash out your differences in private. In your discussions, resist dominating or being dominated, but be willing to hear the other viewpoint and compromise or give in where appropriate. Come up with a plan you can both live with. Consult with each other frequently to keep in sync.

I want to say something about the role of fathers in these challenging situations. It is my experience (granted, a gross generalization) that typically the mother is more emotionally distraught than the father and, as a result, pushes harder to treat the situation as a crisis requiring drastic action. Very often the mother, in her anxiety, is more willing than the father to follow the recommendations of the experts, without reservation—no matter how extensive, expensive, disruptive to the rest of the family, or dubious, those recommendations might be. "You're not getting it," she tells her husband. "We should do *everything* we can to help Gina. If we don't do what the doctors are telling us to do, the results could be disastrous. We can't afford to make a mistake!"

Again, in my experience, it is generally the father (who, we should remember, loves his child as much as his wife does) who expresses reservations. Sometimes these reservations are based on ignorance, shame, resentment, or bias against the culture of therapy. But, just as often, they are based on a sensible, real-life understanding of human psychology. The father's desire to treat the problem using the least invasive means comes from a good and loving place: he wants to respect and build upon the child's innate strengths while preserving her sense of herself as a psychologically healthy young adult. The danger, as many fathers see it, is that—with the well-meaning collusion of the therapeutic community—his child will come to see herself as a damaged adolescent and give up trying to become a productive adult.

It's true that sometimes the father (or occasionally the mother) is simply unenlightened and needs to be persuaded to overcome his prejudices and get with the program. And it's also true that very often the mother is more "psychologically minded," more up to date on the latest psychotherapeutic trends, more involved with the day-to-day problems of her children, more convinced of the merits of her point of view, and more supported by expert opinion. But *sometimes*, all those conditions notwithstanding, the father's incremental, minimalist, even "tough love" approach is right for the situation. The father's reasonable viewpoint should not be derided or dismissed out of hand simply because it's "unsophisticated" or takes cost into consideration. (My admonition to respect this realistic viewpoint applies as much or more to us therapists as it does to parents.) In my experience with college students—especially those who have never before had trouble in school—the "unsophisticated" approach of the dissenting parent often has as much potential to do good as the no-holds-barred "sophisticated" approach of the consenting parent and, more important, has less potential to do harm.

Needless to say (though I'll say it anyway), it's important to properly treat serious mental illness, substance abuse, and learning disabilities. And, needless to say, it's important to fairly evaluate what the experts are saying, to treat them respectfully, and to err on the side of caution. But *their* patient is *your* child. And, after all due diligence has been exercised, you have to trust your own best judgment. The worst possible outcome would be to transform your children into professional patients—chronic invalids who use their illness to avoid the travails and triumphs of living in the real world, falling permanently behind their peers, ceasing to develop, and refusing to grow up.

With a little patience and circumspection, the crisis will abate, the dust will settle, the reality will get separated from the hype, the true problem will declare itself, the proper course of action will become clear—and peace will reign between parent and child and husband and wife. (Not quite the dawning of the Age of Aquarius, perhaps, but close.)

Dealing with the College

In the course of trying to sort out how to help your child, you'll come in contact with a variety of people from the college, the student health service, and the community of therapists near the campus or back home. The first person you're likely to deal with is one of the college deans. In many cases, she will already have been talking to your child by the time you're brought into the picture. The dean can help you and your child deal with administrative issues (such as disciplinary actions and leaves), contact professors and advisers, locate academic and therapeutic resources on campus, connect with the health service, and give counsel and support. Deans vary in competence and helpfulness, like every other expert, but the office of the dean of students is a good place to start your journey.

Dealing with Therapists

If your child is having problems in college—even garden-variety problems—there's a good chance that at some point she'll enter therapy. Because the correct treatment depends on the correct diagnosis, you should make sure she's been adequately evaluated before she starts. Although most counselors associated with colleges are competent and compassionate, not all student health services or college communities have the resources to deal with every problem. If the problem is a complicated or specialized one, it may make sense to seek an opinion from someone in your hometown who has the specific expertise to deal with it. Because therapists assigned by the college health service sometimes have the dual role—and potential conflict of interest—of treating your kid and evaluating whether he's fit to return to class, seeing an outside therapist during medical leaves of absence will help ensure the inviolability of the treatment.

Your responsibility doesn't end once your child is in treatment. You'll want to keep an eye on his progress. Try to get your child's permission to speak with his therapist on occasion to find out how the therapy is going and give the therapist a little feedback. Reassure him that you won't ask the therapist to divulge things that should be kept confidential or try to manipulate the treatment to your own ends.

One of the best ways to establish contact with the therapist is to meet him jointly with your child so that everything is open and aboveboard. It reassures your child that the therapist isn't telling tales out of school. And it gives you the chance to make sure the therapist is competent, aware of what's really going on, and sane. Being kept in the loop helps you—and it helps *you* help your child.

(Exceptions to the confidentiality rule that governs the patient-therapist relationship are serious risk to the patient—such as suicide or dangerous lack of self-care—or serious risk to another person—such as homicide or reckless endangerment. These emergencies require of the therapist a duty to intervene, to protect the patient or other people, that supersedes the important but fixable goal of maintaining the therapeutic alliance.)

If the therapist refuses to talk to you when it's important for her to do so (i.e., when you're rightly concerned and your child hasn't expressly forbidden you to contact the therapist), you should seriously consider whether the therapy is likely to be helpful. Most experienced therapists know how to handle parent contact with discretion and respect while making their patient feel comfortable that no harmful confidences will be divulged.

Your presence on the scene establishes two important facts: 1. that your child has a loving, concerned, and supportive family—as distinct from an angry, intrusive, or negligent one—and 2. that you have a relationship with your child that predates his current relationships, including the one with his therapist, and that *your* relationship, for all its ups and downs, will persist throughout his life. It's important that you and your college-age child—and all the people trying to help him—know that you have a prior and ongoing claim to his respect, consideration, and, yes, love. This does not require you to be adversarial. Every therapist I know tries to do her best and endeavors to put the interests of her patients foremost. But therapists, whatever their level of expertise, can be mistaken. The thing that distinguishes good therapists from therapists who are less good is the willingness to listen to their patients (and sometimes the patient's loved ones) and modify their understanding and approach accordingly.

TAKING THE LONG VIEW

When your child is suffering, the hardest thing to do is to try taking the long view. The advantage you have over your kid is that you've lived long enough to know that "this too shall pass." The disadvantage you have is that you've lived long enough to know that occasionally it doesn't. It's particularly hard for you to take the long view because, to a disturbing degree, your child's fate is out of your control. It's in his hands, not yours. But trying to take the long view is important. It defuses the atmosphere of disappointment and gloom, introduces a sense of proportion and hope, and tells your child that you have faith in him. Taking the long view shows him that you still believe in his resilience and strength, even if he no longer does.

When you're totally in over your head and the future's not yet clear, it's hard to remember that time will heal most wounds. It's easy to lose perspective, become overwhelmed, and give in to despair. If your anxiety or depression gets too much to handle, seek help yourself. But try to step back from the immediate feelings and think about the crises you've been through in *your* life. Did you survive them? Did you learn and grow from them? Did your failures and losses not make you wiser and more compassionate than your successes and triumphs? Did the challenges you confronted in your life not help to make you *you*?

I hope the answer to those questions is yes. But even if it isn't, with your help, the answer can still be yes for your child.

BRAND AND GENERIC NAMES OF DRUGS

Adderall = mixed salts of
amphetamine
Advil PM = ibuprofen plus
diphenhydramine
Ambien = zolpidem
Ativan = lorazepam
Benadryl = diphenhydramine
Dalmane = flurazepam
Dexedrine = dextroamphetamine
Effexor = venlafaxine
Haldol = haloperidal
Klonopin = clonazepam
Lamictal = lamotrigine
Lexapro = escitalopram

Lunesta = eszopiclone
Paxil = paroxetine
Restoril = temazepam
Risperdal = risperidone
Ritalin = methylphenidate
Seroquel = quetiapine
Sonata = zaleplon
Thorazine = chlorpromazine
Tofranil = imipramine
Tylenol PM = acetaminophen plus
diphenhydramine
Valium = diazepam
Xanax = alprazolam
Zoloft = sertraline

Index